Atlas of Mandibular and Maxillary Reconstruction with the Fibula Flap

Giorgio De Santis • Peter G. Cordeiro
Luigi Chiarini
Editors

Atlas of Mandibular and Maxillary Reconstruction with the Fibula Flap

A step-by-step approach

Springer

Editors
Giorgio De Santis
Department of Plastic and Reconst. Surgery
University Hospital of Modena
Modena
Italy

Peter G. Cordeiro
Plastic and Reconstructive Surgery Service
Memorial Sloan Kettering Cancer Center
New York
USA

Luigi Chiarini
Chief of Cranio-maxillo-facial Surgery Unit
University Hospital of Modena
Modena
Italy

ISBN 978-3-030-10682-9 ISBN 978-3-030-10684-3 (eBook)
https://doi.org/10.1007/978-3-030-10684-3

Library of Congress Control Number: 2019933357

This Springer imprint is published by the registered company Springer Nature Switzerland AG
The registered company address is: Gewerbestrasse 11, 6330 Cham, Switzerland

To all my head and neck cancer patients who have inspired, challenged, and motivated me to strive to provide them with the best possible outcomes in reconstruction. I remain constantly amazed by their courage, fortitude, optimism, humor, and grace even under the most challenging and difficult circumstances. To my mentors, colleagues, fellows, residents, and medical students who have contributed in myriad ways to my own education over the past three decades. To my parents who fostered my diverse interests and always encouraged me to make a difference. Finally, to my wife Carolyn and children Christina, Catherine, and Andrew who have provided me with unrelenting love and support; they have graciously sacrificed their time spent with me so that I could follow my career path and passion as an academic surgeon, in the field of reconstructive surgery.

Peter G. Cordeiro, MD, FACS

Preface

The advent of microsurgery in the 1980s dramatically expanded the options for reconstructing defects of the lower and upper jaws, providing the reconstructive surgeon with a wider choice of flaps of skin, soft tissue, and bone. Osteocutaneous free flaps to restore segmental bony defects include the iliac crest, scapula, radius, and fibula, which have radically improved aesthetic and functional outcomes in the ensuing decades. Advantages and disadvantages of each donor site relate to the quality and extent of bone and its ability to be osteotomized and shaped, as well as the amount of soft tissue and skin.

The fibula flap has emerged as the most versatile and most commonly used in jaw reconstruction due to the excellent quantity and quality of bone. The fibula provides 30–35 cm of straight bone that is well vascularized due to intraosseous and periosteal blood supply. The segmental blood supply from the peroneal artery allows for multiple osteotomies without devascularizing individual segments, which permits the reconstructive surgeon to create three-dimensional contours of the missing mandibular and maxillary segments. The thickness of the bone, the bicortical nature, and width (1–2 cm) also allow for the use of osseointegrated implants that maximize functional outcomes, primarily mastication.

The fibula flap has other excellent advantages. The donor site is well removed from the head and neck, which allows for simultaneous dissection of the flap during resection. A single- or double-skin island can be harvested with the bone to include a large portion of the lateral surface area of the leg. This skin can be used to resurface the external skin of the face and neck, provide intraoral lining, close palatal defects, and maximize mobility of the tongue. The skin has a moderate amount of soft tissue that can provide volume in large defects. The flexor hallucis longus muscle can be harvested with the flap and used to fill in dead space in the submental region, cheek, and maxillary sinus. The peroneal artery with its venae comitantes can reliably provide a long pedicle with a large diameter, which maximizes microsurgical success. The pedicle can be lengthened by moving the design of the flap more distally on the leg.

We have focused this book on the use of the fibula flap in reconstruction of the upper and lower jaws because of its great utility and its overwhelming popularity as the first choice for reconstructing a majority of the segmental defects. As the book is an atlas, we have used high-quality photos of illustrative cases to demonstrate technical details and applications of the flap to a variety of defects. We have used the Cordeiro classification systems for defects of the mandible and maxilla because we felt these to be the simplest but most comprehensive classification of the most commonly seen defects after resection. We have included chapters that address dissection of the fibula and reconstruction of the neomandible and neomaxilla, both with traditional templates and virtual surgical planning, as well as sections on indications for reconstruction, preoperative imaging, methods of fixation, osseointegration, postoperative functional assessments, and secondary procedures.

As reconstructive surgeons, we are dedicated to improving the lives of our patients by providing the best care and maximal aesthetic and functional restoration. We hope that this book will help the reader gain a better understanding of how to conceptually and technically approach the challenges of mandibular and maxillary reconstruction.

New York, USA Peter G. Cordeiro
Modena, Italy Giorgio De Santis
Modena, Italy Luigi Chiarini

Contents

Part I

Classification System

Classification System for Mandibulectomy Defects

Peter G. Cordeiro

The mandible, a U-shaped bony structure with posterior vertical extensions, establishes the height, width, and projection of the lower face. The arch of the mandible and the body are the primary teeth-bearing portions, while the ascending ramus with condyles articulates with the skull base posteriorly, which allows for critical functions such as speech and mastication. The bone of the mandible abuts multiple soft-tissue structures that are equally essential to both function and form: anteriorly, the chin, lips, and oral commissures; laterally, the external cheek and intraoral lining; posteriorly, the pharyngeal pillars; and medially, the floor of the mouth and the tongue. Resection of cancers that occur in this region can create not just bony defects but also loss of the surrounding soft-tissue components. Thus, a classification system for mandibular defects must also address the soft-tissue defects. The Cordeiro classification system consists of 13 primary types of defects; the algorithms to approach reconstruction of these defects can vary in the hands of different surgeons, but the reconstructive options generally need to address the specific defect.

Mandibulectomy Defect Classification System

The mandibulectomy defect classification system consists of a Roman numeral, a subdividing letter, and, in subcases, a subcategory number.

The *Roman numeral* (*I*, *II*, *III*) describes the bony defect.

Type I defects involve the anterior arch, which always includes the symphysis but may also include one or both parasymphyses (Fig. 1).

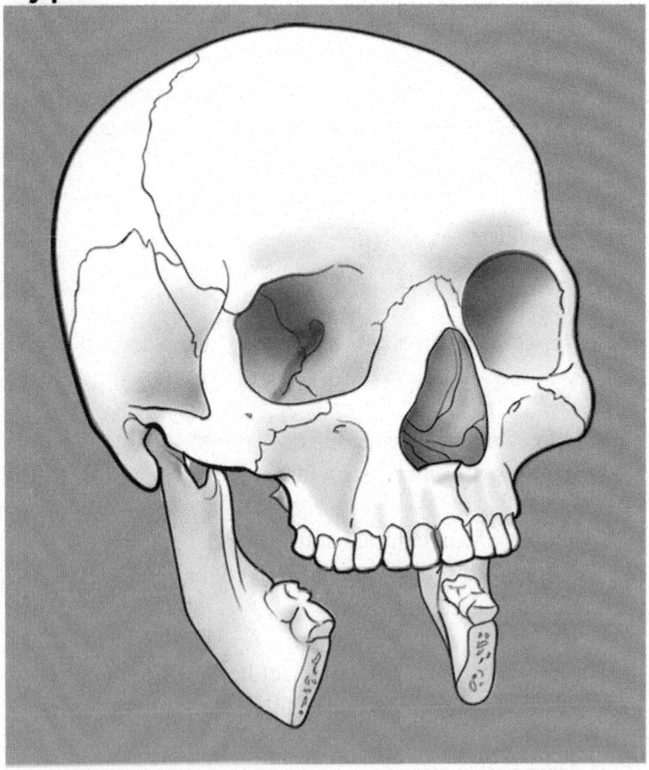

Fig. 1 Type I bony defect, anterior

Type II defects involve the hemimandible and always include a portion of the body, the angle, and the ascending ramus (with or without the condyle) (Fig. 2).

Type III defects are lateral defects that involve one or two out of three of the following components: the ascending ramus, angle, or body (Fig. 3).

A letter (*A*, *B*, *C*, *D*) describes the quality of the soft-tissue defect and involvement of any combination of the skin, subcutaneous tissue, muscle, intraoral structures, and mucosal lining.

P. G. Cordeiro (✉)
Plastic and Reconstructive Surgery Service, Memorial Sloan Kettering Cancer Center, Weill Medical College of Cornell University, New York, NY, USA
e-mail: cordeirp@MSKCC.ORG

G. De Santis et al. (eds.), *Atlas of Mandibular and Maxillary Reconstruction with the Fibula Flap*,
https://doi.org/10.1007/978-3-030-10684-3_1

Type II

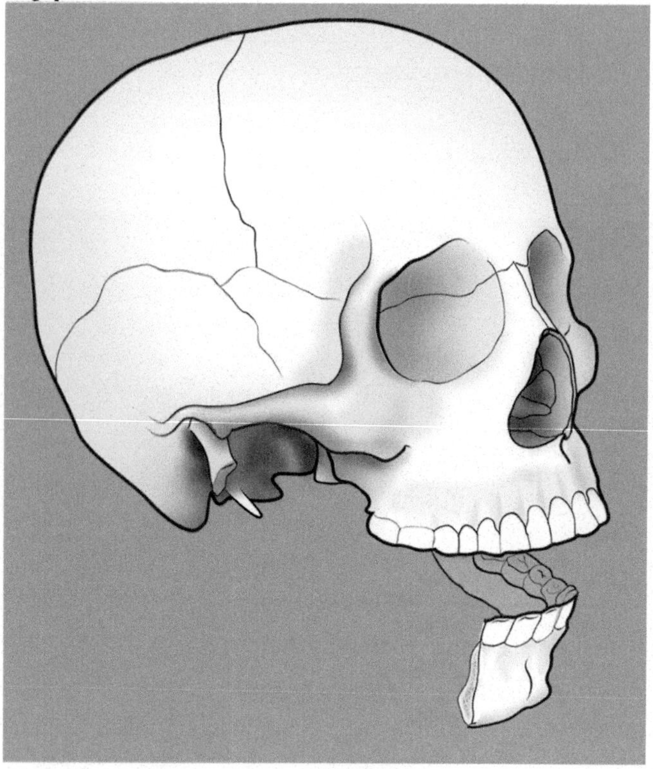

Fig. 2 Type II bony defect, hemimandible

Type III

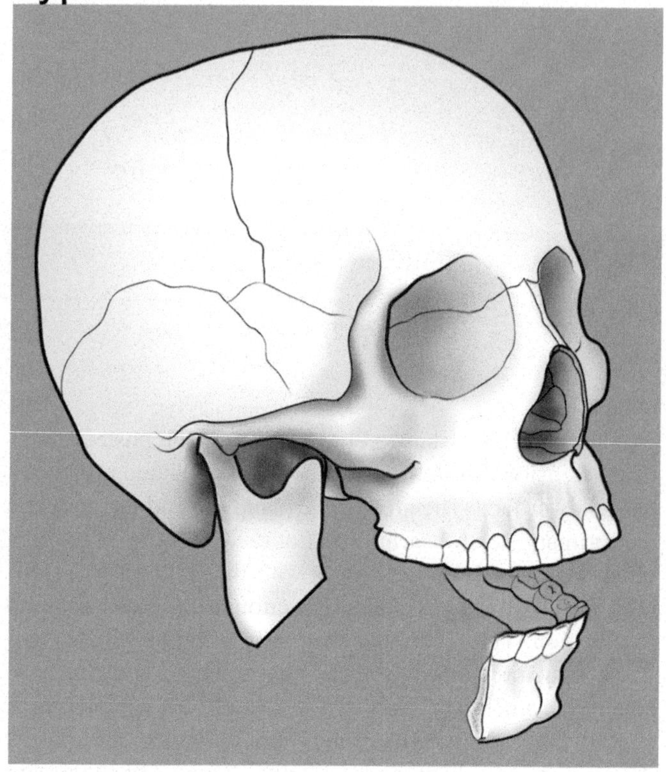

Fig. 3 Type III bony defect, lateral

- *A* denotes no soft-tissue defect.
- *B* denotes intraoral structure and/or mucosal lining defect.
- *C* denotes a skin/external soft-tissue defect only.
- *D* denotes a through-and-through or both intraoral structures/lining and skin defect.

The extent of the intraoral defect has been found to commonly dictate the reconstruction algorithm for type II hemimandibular defects; therefore, a *subclassification of B1 and B2* is described.

Based on five zones of intraoral structures that include the buccal mucosa, floor of mouth, palate, tongue, and pharynx.

- Excision of *two or fewer* intraoral zones is designated *B1*.
- Excision of *three or more* intraoral zones is designated *B2*.

Thus, a classification system of 13 principal zones is described (Fig. 4).

- *IA, IB, IC, ID*
- *IIA, IIB1, IIB2, IIC, IID*
- *IIIA, IIIB, IIIC, IIID*

The algorithm to reconstruct each type of mandibular defect must first consider the location of the resected bone and then the required soft-tissue deficits.

Fig. 4 Mandibulectomy defect classification system

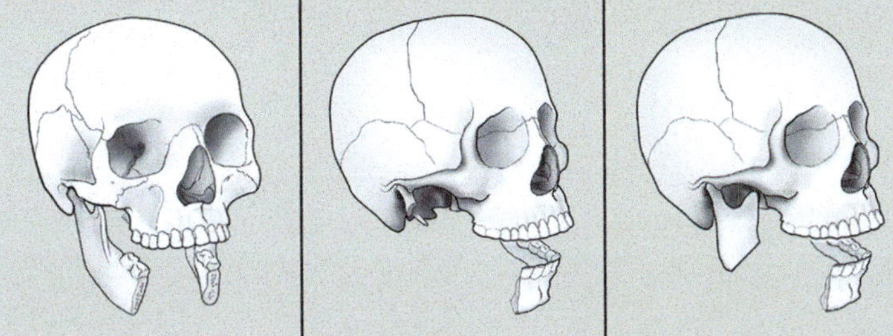

Soft tissue defect	Bony defect: Anterior	Bony defect: Hemimandible	Bony defect: Lateral
None	IA	IIA	IIIA
Intraoral only	IB	IIB1 ≤ 2 zones IIB2 ≥ 3 zones	IIIB
Skin only	IC	IIC	IIIC
Intraoral + skin	ID	IID	IIID

Further Reading

Cordeiro PG, Henderson PW, Matros E. A 20-year experience with 202 segmental mandibulectomy defects: a defect classification system, algorithm for flap selection and surgical outcomes. Plast Reconstr Surg. 2018;141(4):571e–81e.

Cordeiro PG, Hidalgo DA. Conceptual considerations in mandibular reconstruction. Clin Plastic Surg. 1995;22:61–9.

Classification System for Maxillectomy Defects

Peter G. Cordeiro

The two maxillary bones contribute to creating a major portion of the midfacial skeleton, which is critical to both form and function in the midface. The maxilla is essentially a tetrahedron, with the roof of the maxilla supporting the globe and orbital contents; the floor of the maxilla being the hard palate; the maxillary arch being the tooth-bearing component; and the four vertical walls of the maxilla contributing to maintaining the height and projection of the midface and the medial wall forming the lateral walls of the nasal cavity (Fig. 1).

The maxilla is in close contiguity to multiple critical soft tissue areas, and cancer resections will often include resection of this soft tissue in conjunction with certain walls of the maxilla. These areas include the external skin and soft tissues, as well as muscles of the midface, the lips/oral commissure, nose/nasal lining, and orbital contents extending up to the cranial base.

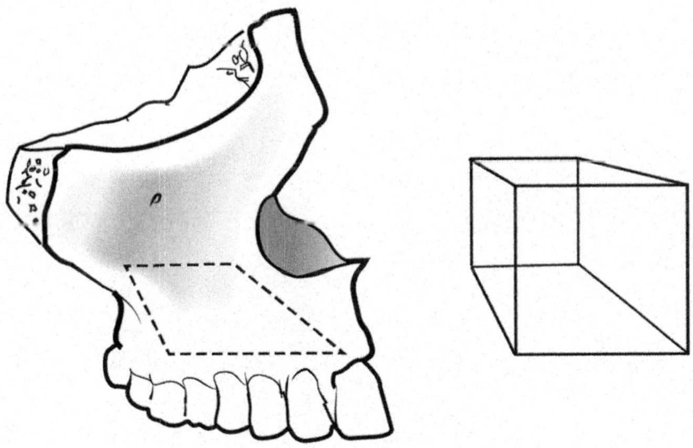

Fig. 1 The maxilla is conceptually a tetrahedron

P. G. Cordeiro (✉)
Plastic and Reconstructive Surgery Service, Memorial Sloan Kettering Cancer Center, Weill Medical College of Cornell University, New York, NY, USA
e-mail: cordeirp@MSKCC.ORG

Maxillectomy Defect Classification System

The maxillectomy defect classification system follows the most common patterns of resection of the bony structure of the maxilla plus/minus the contiguous soft tissues. There are six principal types of maxillectomy defects: *I*, *IIA*, *IIB*, *IIIA*, *IIIB*, and *IV*.

Type I: Limited Maxillectomy Defects

These most commonly include one or two walls of the maxilla, usually the anterior and medial walls, often the skin/soft tissues of the cheek overlying the maxilla, and occasionally critical structures such as the lips, nose, and eyelids (Fig. 2).

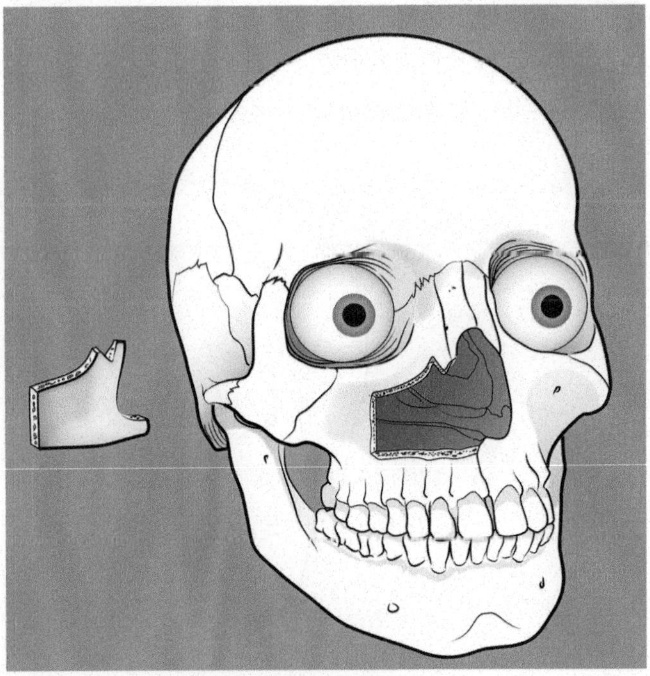

Fig. 2 Type I maxillectomy or limited defects

G. De Santis et al. (eds.), *Atlas of Mandibular and Maxillary Reconstruction with the Fibula Flap*,
https://doi.org/10.1007/978-3-030-10684-3_2

Type II: Subtotal Maxillectomy Defects

These defects include resection of the lower five walls of the maxilla, which include the palate and dentoalveolar arch but leave the orbital floor intact.

Type IIA defects include less than 50% of the arch of the maxilla and do not extend past the midline (Fig. 3).

Type IIB defects involve greater than 50% of the maxillary arch and extend past the midline. Many of these defects can include bilateral maxillae and involve the entire arch (Fig. 4).

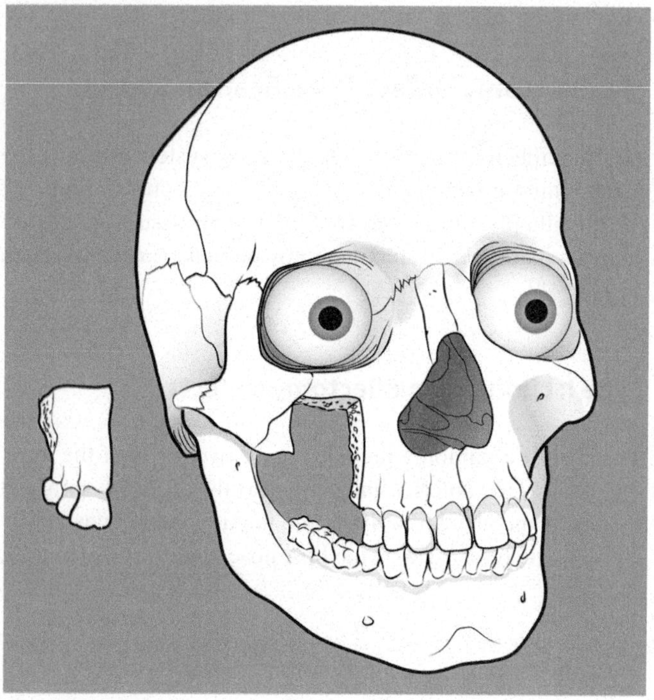

Fig. 3 Type IIA subtotal maxillectomy defect

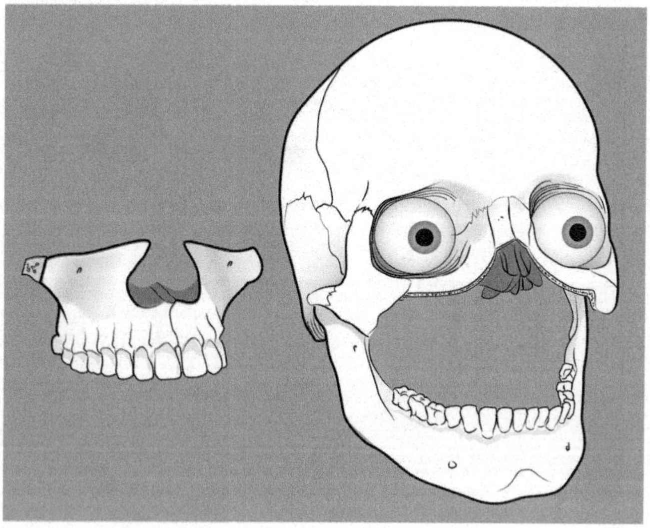

Fig. 4 Type IIB subtotal maxillectomy defect

Type III: Total Maxillectomy Defects

These defects include resection of all six walls of the maxilla, including the floor of the orbit and palate/alveolar arch, and may or may not include resection of the orbital contents.

Type IIIA defects involve resection of all six walls of the maxilla, including the floor of the orbit but sparing the orbital contents (Fig. 5).

Type IIIB defects involve resection of all six walls of the maxilla, including exenteration of the orbital contents (Fig. 6).

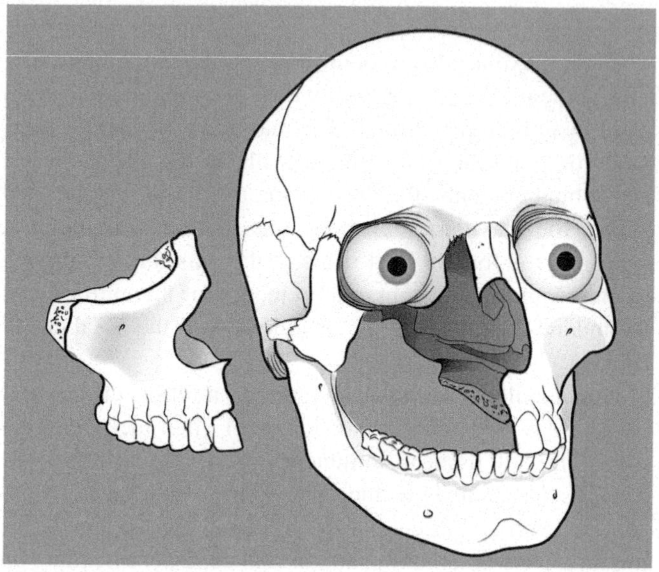

Fig. 5 Type IIIA total maxillectomy defect sparing the orbital contents

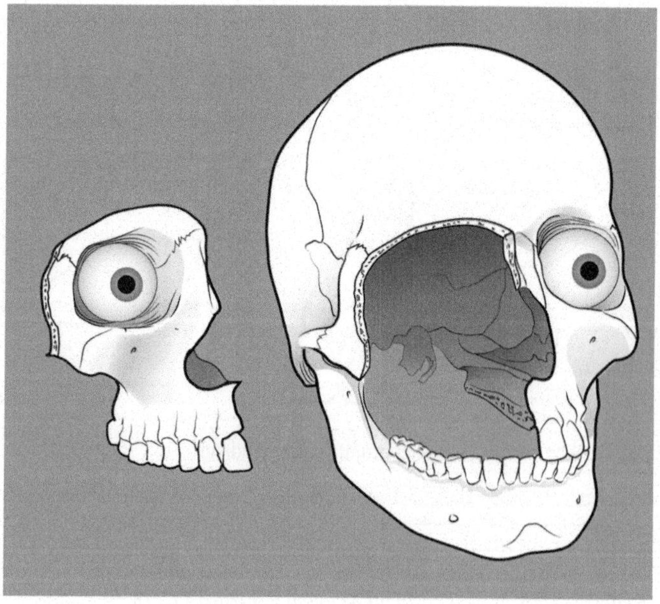

Fig. 6 Type IIIB total maxillectomy defect including the orbital contents

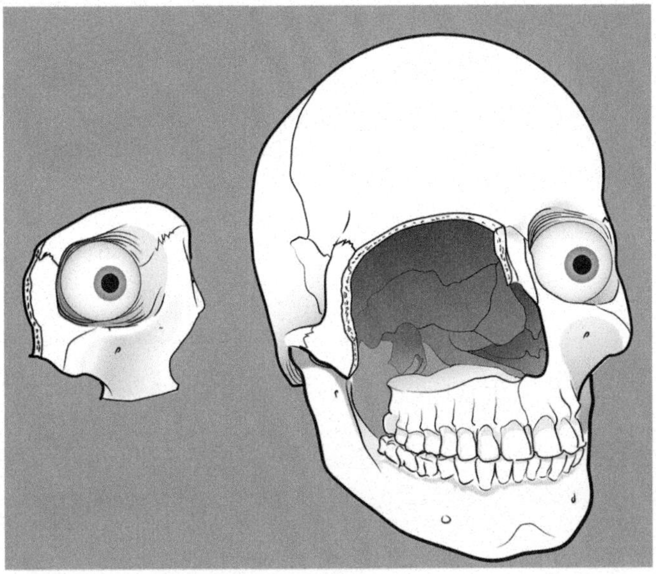

Fig. 7 Type IV orbitomaxillectomy defect

Type IV: Orbitomaxillectomy Defects

These defects involve resection of the upper maxilla/floor of orbit and the orbital contents (Fig. 7).

The algorithms for reconstruction of the various types of maxillectomy defects vary from surgeon to surgeon, but the conceptual approach addresses the bony deficits as well as the soft tissue, skin, and oral/nasal deficits.

Further Reading

Cordeiro PG, Chen CM. A 15-year review of midface reconstruction after total and subtotal maxillectomy: part I. algorithm and outcomes. Plast Reconstr Surg. 2012;129:124–36.

Cordeiro PG, Santamaria E. A classification system and algorithm for reconstruction of maxillectomy and midfacial defects. Plast Reconstr Surg. 2000;105:2331–46.

McCarthy CM, Cordeiro PG. Microvascular reconstruction of oncologic defects of the midface. Plast Reconstr Surg. 2010;126(6):1947–59.

Part II

Technique and Examples

The Fibula Osteocutaneous Free Flap: Surgical Approach

Peter G. Cordeiro

The fibula is the workhorse osseous flap for mandibular and maxillary reconstruction. It provides a significant amount—up to 30 cm in length—of good-quality cortical bone. The fibula flap may be harvested as a purely osseus flap or be combined with muscle, fascia, and skin to provide soft-tissue elements that may be required for reconstruction. The flap has an excellent pedicle based on the peroneal artery and venae comitantes, with large-diameter vessels up to 3–4 mm. A significantly sized skin paddle designed on the lateral leg can be as large as 10–12 cm in the anteroposterior dimension and 20–25 cm in the longitudinal dimension. The flexor hallucis longus muscle can be taken in its entirety to provide excellent soft-tissue fill. The bone has both an intraosseous blood supply and a periosteal blood supply that allows for the ability to perform multiple osteotomies, which can be shaped to create the various contours of the mandible or the maxilla. The highly reliable fibula flap can be dissected simultaneously with the resection for trauma or disease in the head and neck, significantly decreasing operating time.

Operative Technique: Surface Markings and Skin Island Design

The skin island is always centered over the septum between the lateral and posterior compartment muscles. This septum can be identified by palpating the posterior border of the fibula and drawing a line along the posterior border. As long as the skin island is centered over this septum, there should be an excellent blood supply, particularly in the distal two-thirds of the leg, where the main septocutaneous perforators lie. The transverse dimension of the skin island is relatively small; if less than 3–4 cm, it is usually closed primarily, making this an excellent donor site. For wider dimensions, a skin graft is placed on the muscle after removal of the flap. It is useful to draw the approximate course of the superficial peroneal nerve, which crosses the fibula 2–3 cm below the fibula head. It is also useful to draw the approximate location of the pedicle connection to the bone (Fig. 1).

Anterior Dissection of the Skin, the Lateral Septum, and the Lateral/Anterior Muscle Compartments

After partially exsanguinating the leg with a tourniquet, the dissection is started anteriorly. The incision is carried through the subcutaneous tissues, and the skin and fascia are dissected off the lateral compartment muscles (Fig. 2). Great care is taken to avoid injuring the septum, which carries the blood supply to the skin. Sometimes, there are obvious, large septocutaneous perforators within the septum; if these are not visible, as long as the septum is not injured by the cautery, there is usually adequate blood supply to the skin (Fig. 3).

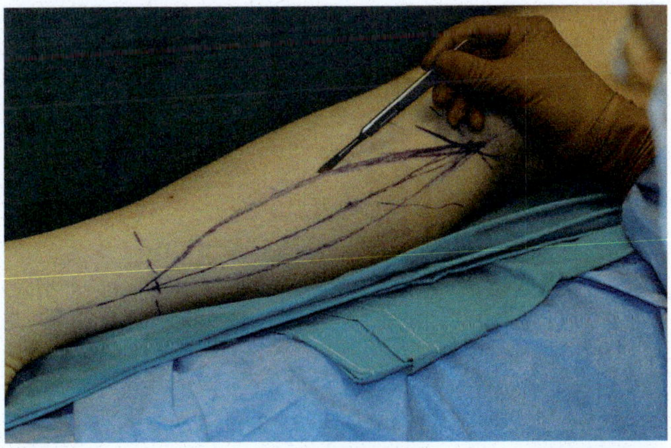

Fig. 1 Design of skin island and incision on the left lower lateral extremity

P. G. Cordeiro (✉)
Plastic and Reconstructive Surgery Service, Memorial Sloan Kettering Cancer Center, Weill Medical College of Cornell University, New York, NY, USA
e-mail: cordeirp@MSKCC.ORG

G. De Santis et al. (eds.), *Atlas of Mandibular and Maxillary Reconstruction with the Fibula Flap*,
https://doi.org/10.1007/978-3-030-10684-3_3

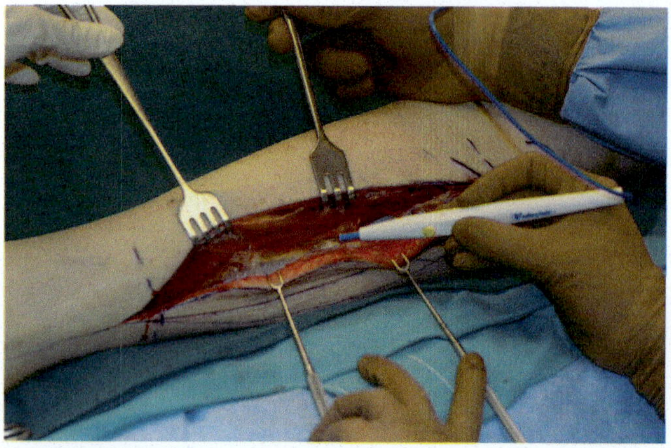

Fig. 2 Anterior dissection with elevation of skin island and fascia off the lateral compartment muscles

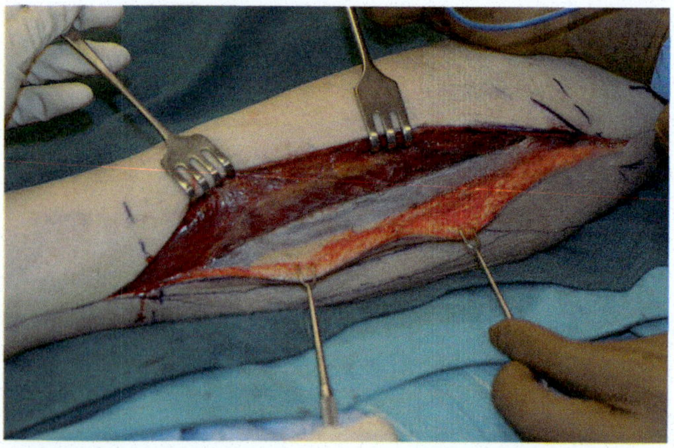

Fig. 3 Skin island dissected off lateral compartment muscles. Note intramuscular septum between lateral and posterior compartment

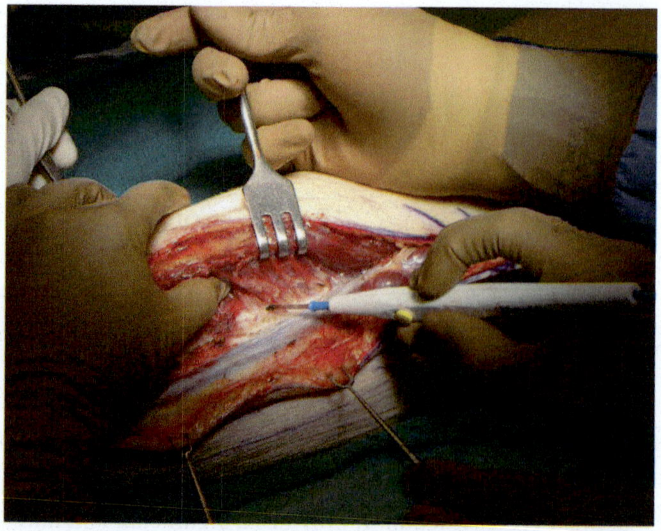

Fig. 4 Lateral compartment muscles dissected off the lateral fibula

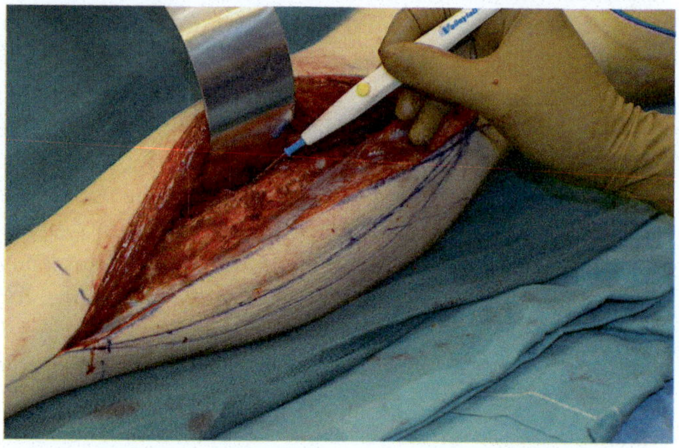

Fig. 5 Completely dissected lateral edge of the fibula with cautery pen used to divide interosseous membrane

Once the dissection reaches the lateral surface of the fibula, the lateral compartment muscles are dissected by leaving a cuff of muscle (2–3 mm) on the bone to avoid injuring the periosteum. Using the surgeon's thumb and retractors on the lateral compartment muscles, the muscle is carefully dissected off the bone (Fig. 4). Within the lateral compartment muscles, caution is taken to avoid branches of the vessels and nerves that enter the muscle.

Once the lateral compartment muscles are dissected, the septum between the lateral and anterior compartment muscles is incised. This septum originates from the anterior surface of the fibula, which is triangular at the apex. Once this septum is incised, the anterior compartment muscles are visible and similarly dissected off the fibula. This is a relatively short distance, and due care is taken to keep the dissection close to the bone while also leaving a small cuff of the muscle. Particular care is exercised to avoid injuring branches of the anterior tibial vessels, which run within the muscle, as well as the anterior tibial nerve. Once this muscle is dissected off the bone, the interosseous membrane is identified and incised across the entirety of the dissection in a distal-to-proximal direction. When incising the interosseous membrane, great caution is taken to avoid injuring the posterior tibial vessels, which run in close contiguity to the bone and to the septum (Fig. 5).

Posterior Dissection of the Skin Island

The posterior skin margin is incised, and special care is taken not to dissect through the septum. To avoid injuring the septum and blood supply to the skin, the septum is palpated by placing the surgeon's fingers directly on the septum anteriorly (Fig. 6).

There are often large perforators from the soleus muscle to the skin island. These usually cannot be preserved,

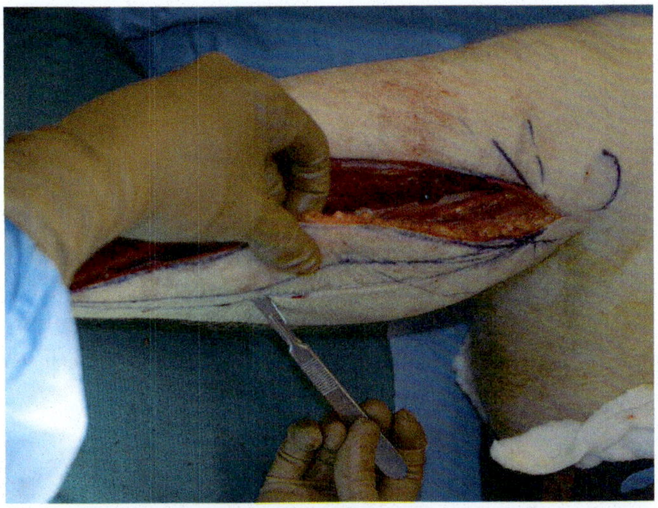

Fig. 6 Posterior skin incision

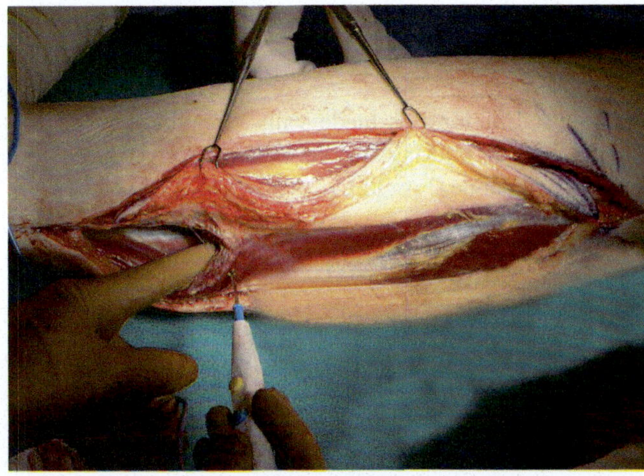

Fig. 8 Separation of the lateral intramuscular septum from the soleus muscle leaving some fibers of the soleus on the septum

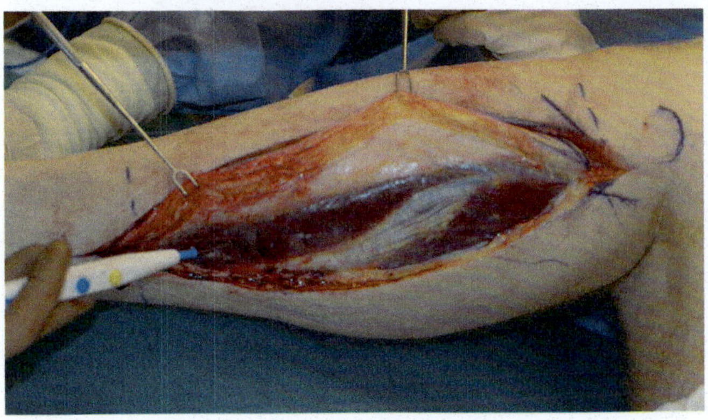

Fig. 7 Skin island elevated off posterior compartment muscles

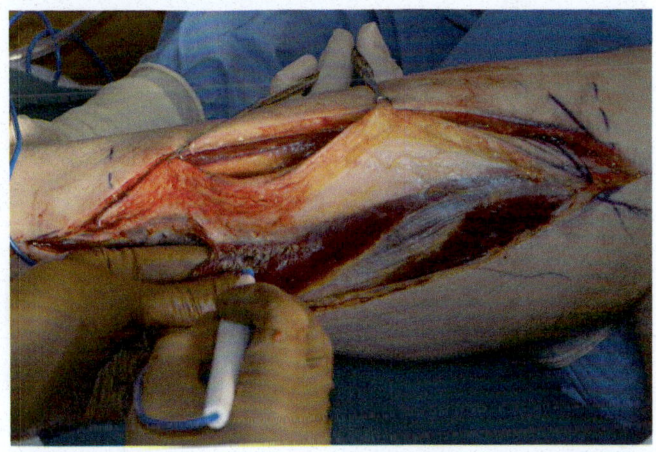

Fig. 9 Continuation of distal to proximal dissection of the soleus muscle off the septum

because they originate from the posterior tibial vessels. They can be safely cauterized or ligated if they are much larger (Fig. 7).

Cautery is used to separate the septum from the soleus. It is preferable to take a small (2–3 mm) cuff of the soleus with the septum to avoid thermal injury to the septum. A distal-to-proximal dissection is best (Fig. 8). More proximally, the main pedicle (the peroneal artery and venae comitantes) becomes obvious, and care is taken to avoid injury to these vessels (Fig. 9).

Once the dissection is carried all the way proximally, caution is exercised to not injure the superficial peroneal nerve, which is within the soft tissues of the proximal leg overlying the fibula. The main pedicle is identified proximally, and the larger perforators from the posterior tibial artery are ligated as they enter the soleus muscle. Once most of the pedicle is identified, the fascia overlying the flexor hallucis longus muscle is incised to allow this muscle to be brought out of the wound (Fig. 10).

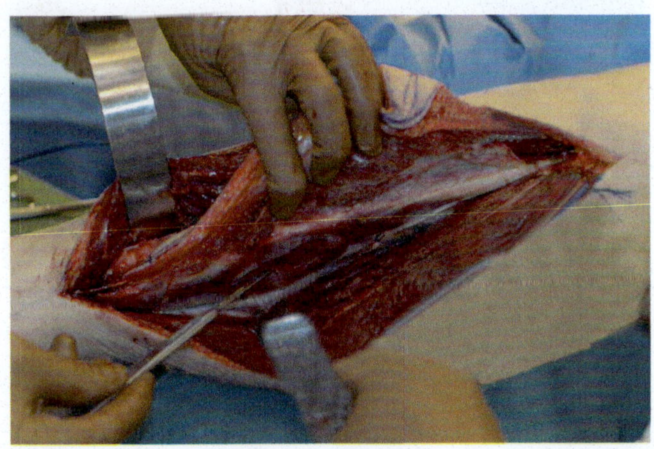

Fig. 10 Fascia over flexor hallucis longus muscle incised. Note main pedicle just posterior to the muscle

Proximal and Distal Osteotomies of the Fibula

The distal osteotomy is made with a sagittal saw. Care is taken to avoid injuring the peroneal vessels that lie just medial to the bone (Fig. 11).

The proximal osteotomy is usually made as high as possible. Even if this portion of the bone is not necessary for the reconstruction, it is helpful to make the osteotomy just below the level of the peroneal nerve and the level where the anterior tibial vessels pierce the interosseus septum as they travel into the anterior compartment. This allows better exposure for dissection of the pedicle. Great care is taken to avoid injuring the nerve and these vessels when making the osteotomy. It is sometimes useful to dissect behind the bone and place a small retractor to avoid injury to the vessels and nerve (Fig. 12).

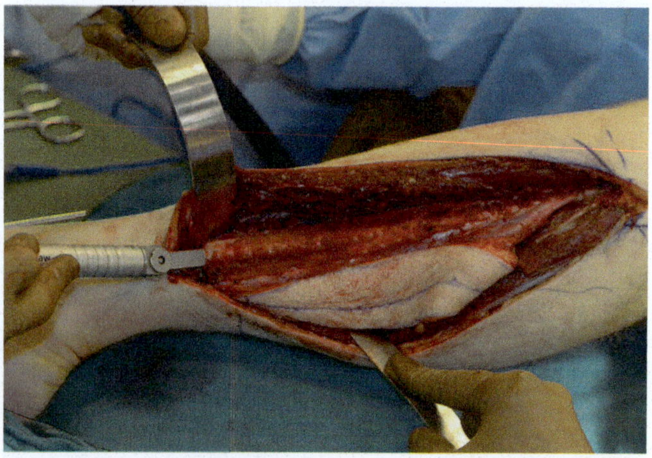

Fig. 11 Distal osteotomy of the fibula

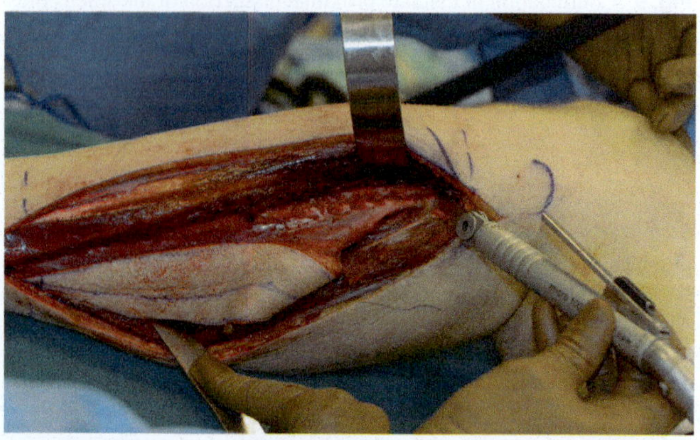

Fig. 12 Proximal osteotomy of the fibula just below the level of the peroneal nerve

Division of the Distal Peroneal Vessels and the Tibialis Posterior Muscle

Once the osteotomies are made, the flap is retracted from the wound, and the distal peroneal vessels and the tibialis posterior muscle are identified (Fig. 13). The tibialis posterior muscle is a bipennate muscle, and the midline raphe is identified. The distal vessels are ligated, which releases the bony segment from the wound (Fig. 14). The flexor hallucis longus muscle is divided, which allows the fibula to be brought out further from the depths of the wound (Fig. 15).

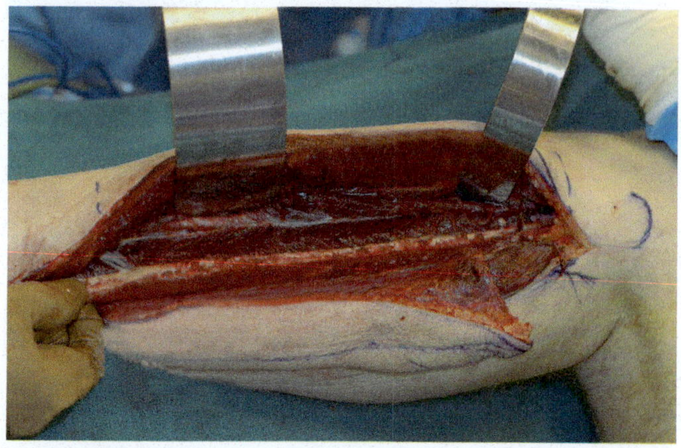

Fig. 13 Osteocutaneous flap retracted out of wound. Note distal peroneal vessels

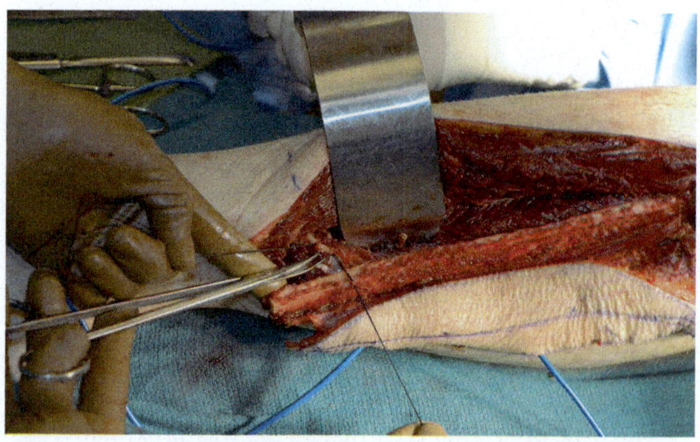

Fig. 14 Ligation and division of distal peroneal vessels

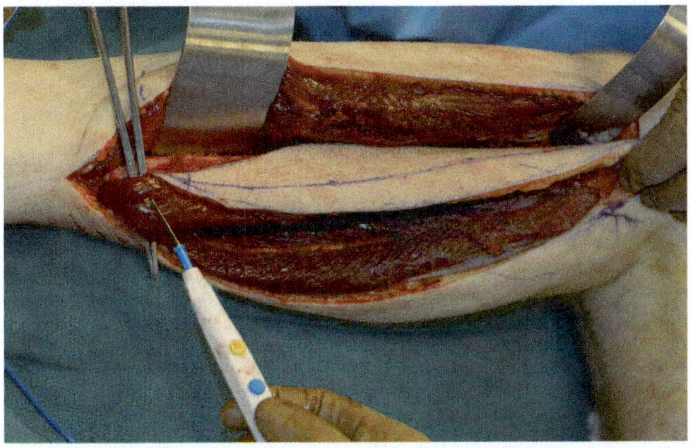

Fig. 15 Division of the distal flexor hallucis longus muscle

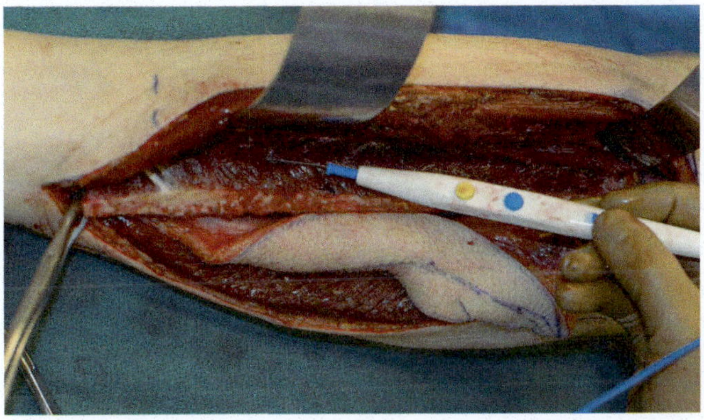

Fig. 16 Cautery pen identifying the bipennate tibialis posterior muscle

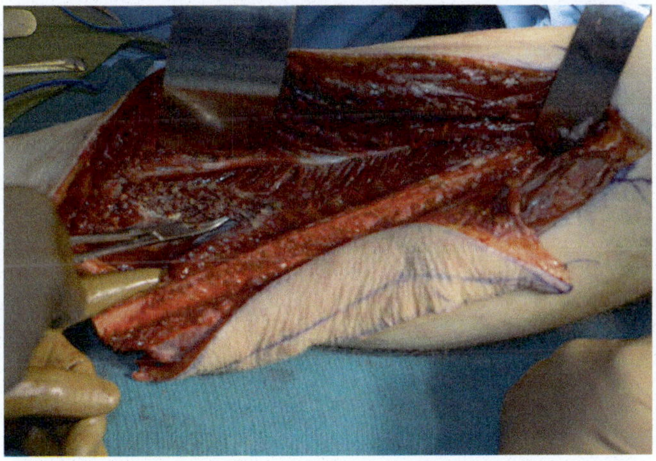

Fig. 17 Division of bipennate tibialis muscle through midline raphe

Dissection of the Main Pedicle

The dissection is carried through the midline raphe (Fig. 16) to preserve the peroneal vessels on the surface of the fibula and the posterior tibial vessels deeper in the wound. The dissection is carried out from distal to proximal (Fig. 17). The tibial nerve lies between the peroneal vessels and the posterior tibial vessels (Fig. 18). The peroneal vessels are dissected to the bifurcation of the posterior tibial and peroneal vessels (Fig. 19). The tourniquet is released, and careful hemostasis is achieved without injuring the anterior and posterior compartment nerves.

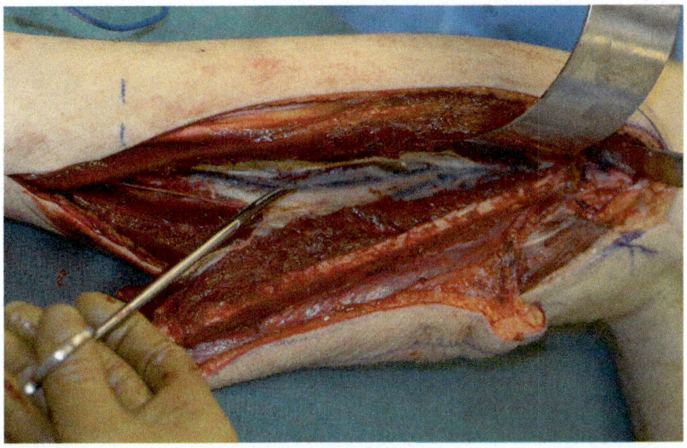

Fig. 18 Final dissection and separation of peroneal vessels from the tibial nerve and posterior tibial vessels medially

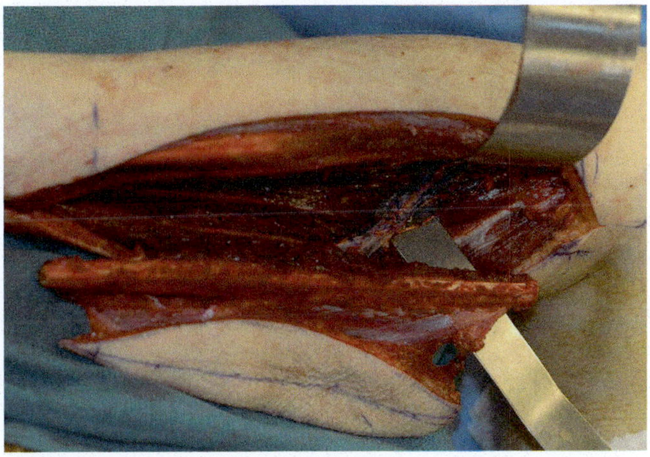

Fig. 19 Osteocutaneous fibula flap with peroneal vessels dissected to the bifurcation of the tibioperoneal trunk

Further Reading

Cordeiro PG, Disa JJ, Hidalgo DA, Hu QY. Reconstruction of the mandible with osseous free flaps: a 10-year experience with 150 consecutive patients. Plast Reconstr Surg. 1999;104:1314–20.

Wallace CG, Tsao CK, Wei FC. Mandibular reconstruction. In: Farhadieh R, Bulstrode N, Cugno S, editors. Plastic and reconstructive surgery: approaches and techniques. Oxford: Wiley-Blackwell; 2015.

Part III

Mandibular and Maxilla Reconstruction

Use of Templates to Perform Osteotomies of the Fibula and to Shape the Neo-mandible or Neomaxilla

Peter G. Cordeiro and Evan Matros

Multiple closing wedge osteotomies of the straight fibula bone are necessary to recreate the three-dimensional shape of the mandible or maxilla. These osteotomies have traditionally been accomplished using templates based upon a preoperative CT scan and lateral cephalogram of the patient. More recently, using a virtual platform, computer-assisted design and modeling in combination with additive printing have been used. Each technique has pros and cons, so it is important for reconstructive surgeons to be familiar with both methods. For most cases, the highly conserved angulation of the parasymphysis, mid-body, and angle enables reliable and efficient use of traditional templates without the added cost or time necessary for virtual surgical planning (VSP). In contrast, for cases where reliable measurement of the specimen cannot be performed because of tumor distortion, or for delayed reconstruction, VSP has inherent advantages. The current chapter describes how to perform osteotomies using either technique.

The use of templates is the traditional, well-established method for performing closing wedge osteotomies to convert a straight, long fibula bone flap into the shape of a mandible. Two templates are usually necessary to establish the osteotomy angles. The first template is made by tracing a 1:1 axial CT scan of the mandible onto an X-ray sheet using the CT section closest to the lower border of the mandible and with the most complete outline of the mandible (Fig. 1). The X-ray sheet can be sterilized and used as a template, but the usual practice is to trace the X-ray sheet onto an acrylic sheet to create a more durable acrylic template. This template provides the angles for parasymphyseal and mid-body osteotomies by converting the slight curvature of the mandibular border into straight lines. The second template is made by tracing a lateral cephalogram onto an X-ray sheet, which is also converted to an acrylic template (Fig. 2). This second template provides the angle of the mandible also by converting the slight curvature within the bone of the mandible into straight lines and a precise angle.

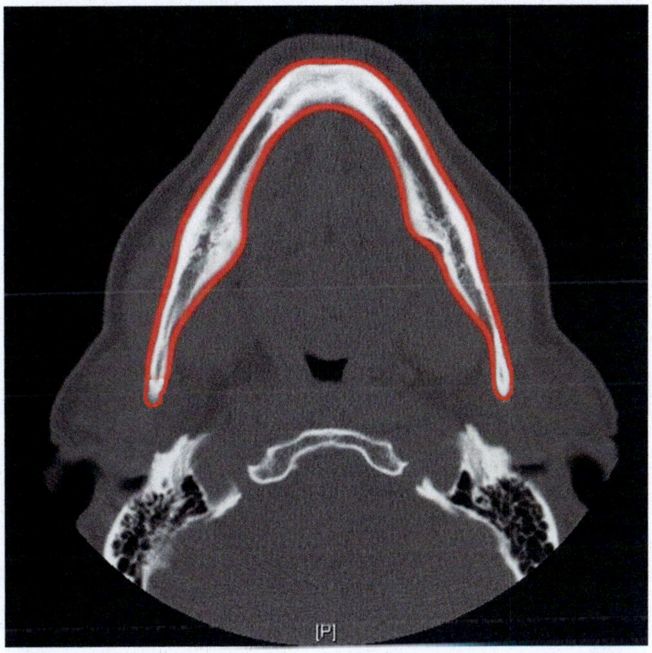

Fig. 1 Template traced from axial CT of mandible

A closing wedge osteotomy at the angle of the mandible is shown (Figs. 1 and 2) to demonstrate how to use the mandibular angle template. The patient has undergone resection of the angle of the mandible. Figures 3 and 4 show the patient after resection and the specimen, respectively. The specimen is saved in order to compare it with the template and final reconstruction (Fig. 5). The condyle is resected and preserved so that it can be transplanted into the fibula if this is oncologically safe (Fig. 6). Once the template is prepared, a straight line is scored on the template bisecting the angle that is needed (Fig. 7). The template is placed along the lower edge of the fibula, and the scored line is transferred onto the fibula

P. G. Cordeiro (✉) · E. Matros
Plastic and Reconstructive Surgery Service, Memorial Sloan Kettering Cancer Center, Weill Medical College of Cornell University, New York, NY, USA
e-mail: cordeirp@MSKCC.ORG; matrose@mskcc.org

G. De Santis et al. (eds.), *Atlas of Mandibular and Maxillary Reconstruction with the Fibula Flap*,
https://doi.org/10.1007/978-3-030-10684-3_4

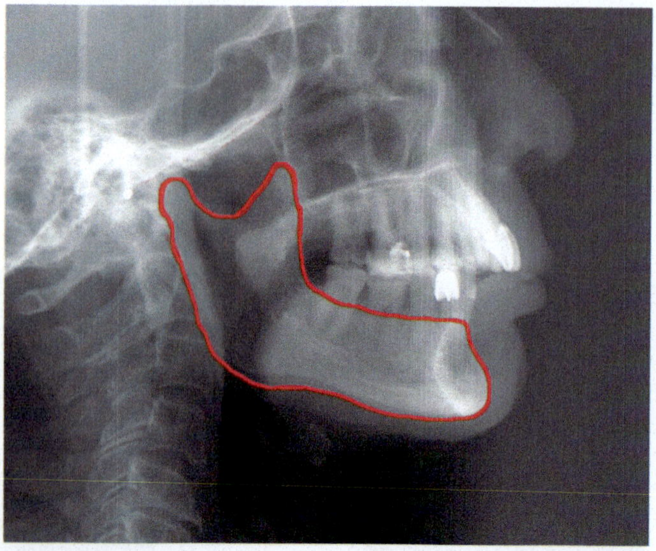

Fig. 2 Template traced from lateral cephalogram

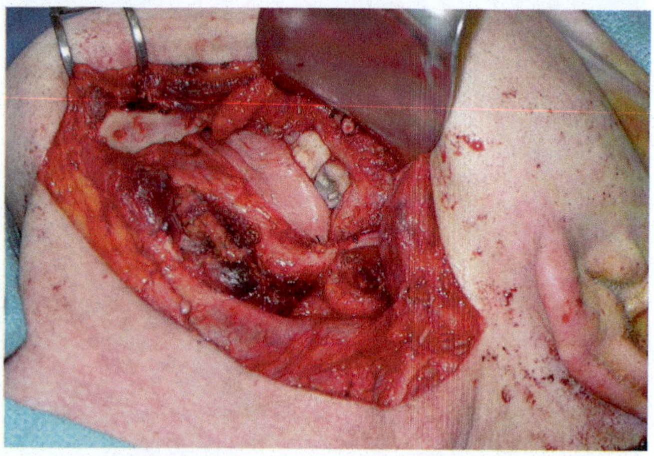

Fig. 3 Left lateral segmental defect of mandible

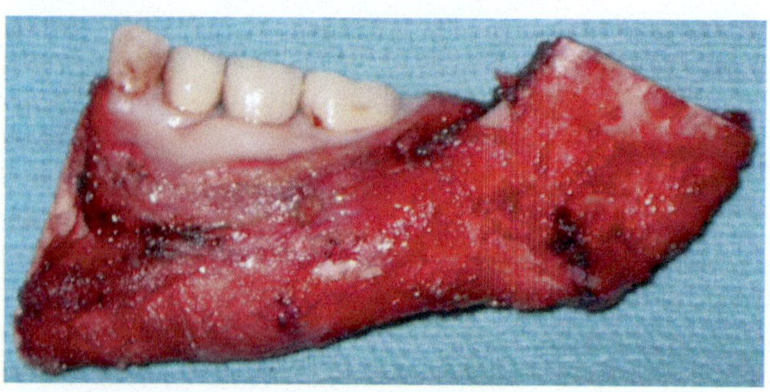

Fig. 4 Resected left hemimandibular specimen

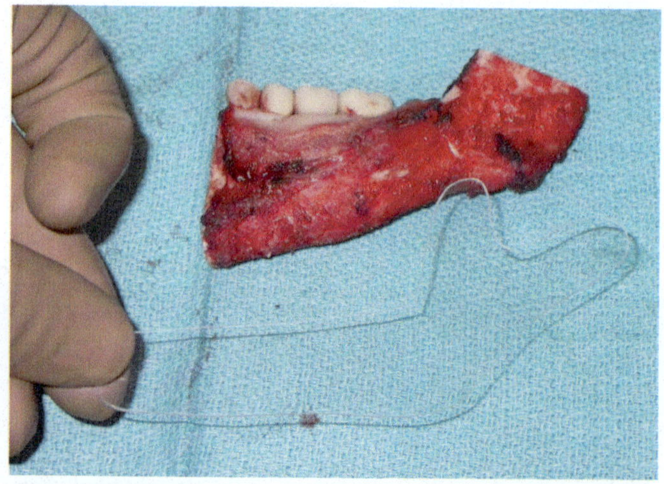

Fig. 5 Acrylic template compared with actual angle of the resected hemimandible

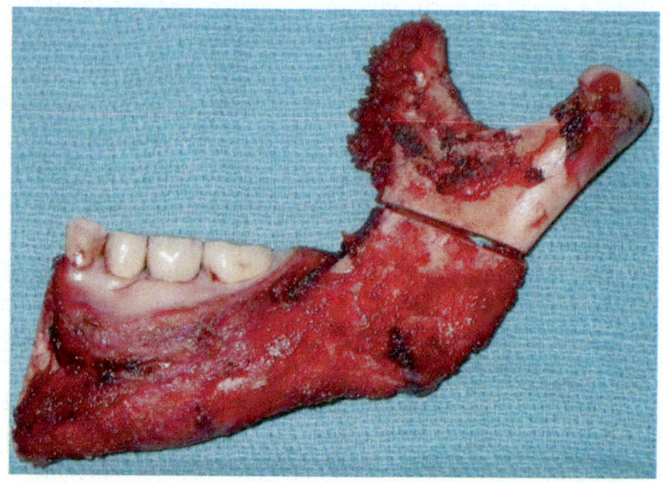

Fig. 6 Specimen transected in subcondylar region to obtain condyle for autotransplantation

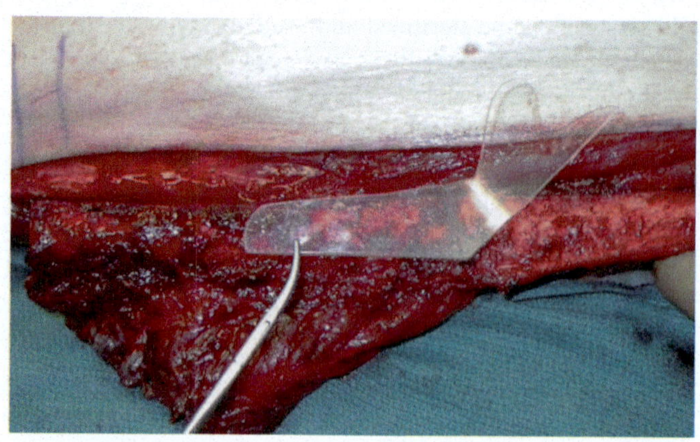

Fig. 7 Template aligned with posterior edge of the fibula

(Fig. 8). The ascending ramus margin of the template is placed along the lower edge of the fibula. The edge of the template that duplicates the body is placed along the lower edge of the fibula, and the same scored line is transferred onto the fibula (Fig. 9). The closing wedge osteotomy is completed using the sagittal saw (Fig. 10). Once these two edges are brought together (Fig. 11), the template is used to finalize this angle to exactly duplicate the angle that is necessary (Fig. 12). The fibula is then rigidly fixed in two planes (Fig. 13).

Using the mandibular arch template, the same process is followed on the fibula in the plane needed to design the closing parasymphyseal and mid-body osteotomies (Fig. 14). Miniplates fixed in two planes are preferred: one along the lateral border of the fibula and the other along the posterior border. However, this same technique could be applied using a larger mandibular reconstruction plate. Compared to the use of reconstruction plate, miniplates provide the greatest accuracy and the lowest profile for the actual fibula to establish the contour of the mandible.

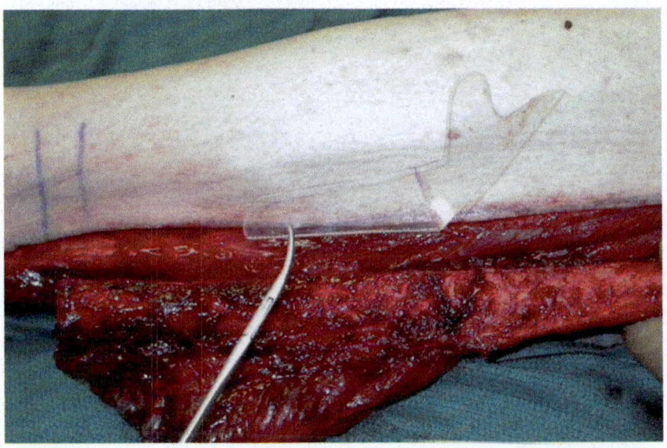

Fig. 8 Template with wedge-shaped osteotomy lines transferred to the fibula

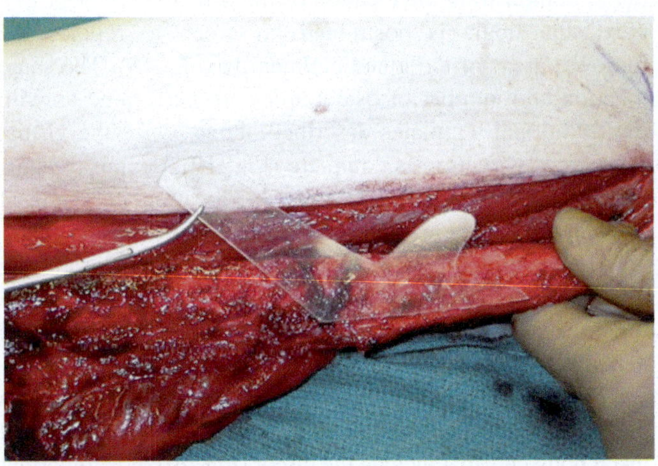

Fig. 9 Template with scored line at angle used to transfer angles of osteotomy

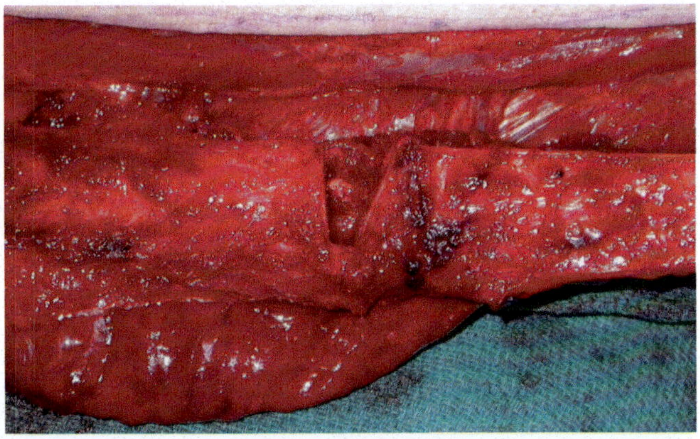

Fig. 10 Completed closing wedge osteotomy of the fibula

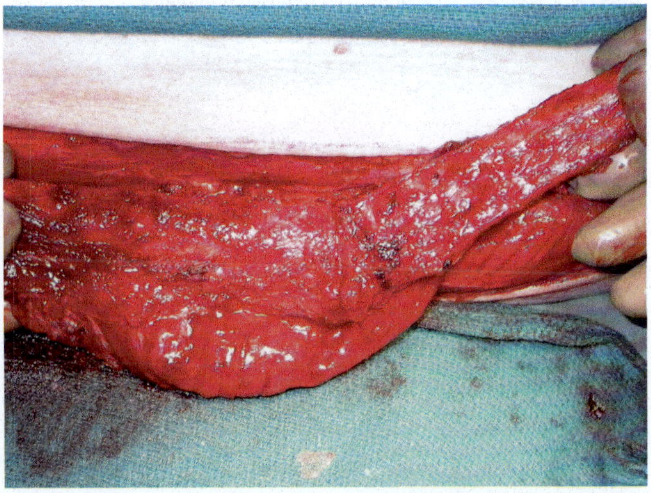

Fig. 11 Edges of osteotomy approximated to recreate angle of mandible

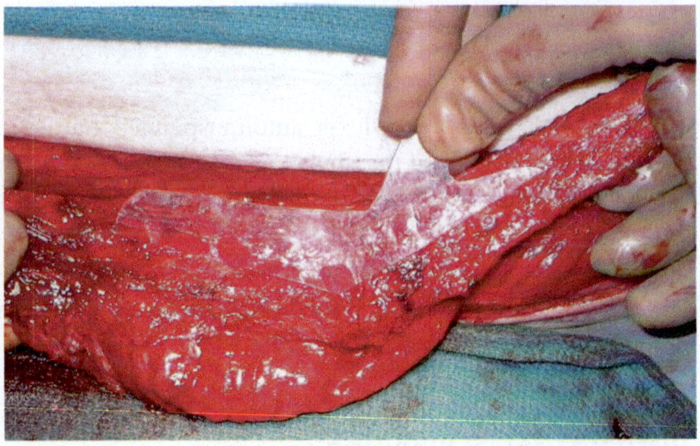

Fig. 12 Template aligned with neo-angle created by osteotomy

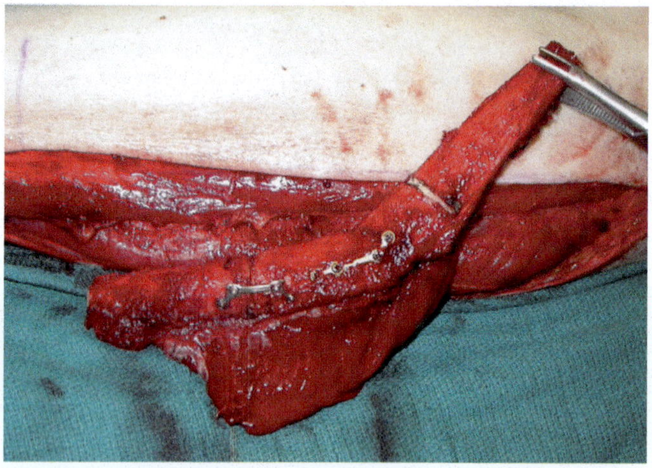

Fig. 13 Fibula rigidly fixated with titanium miniplates

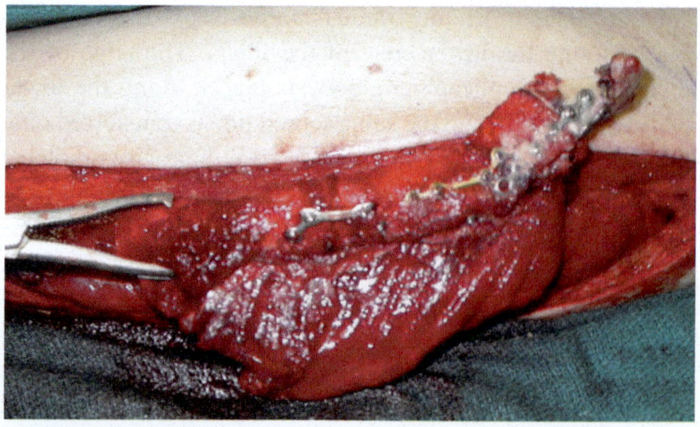

Fig. 15 Condyle autotransplanted into position on neo-mandible

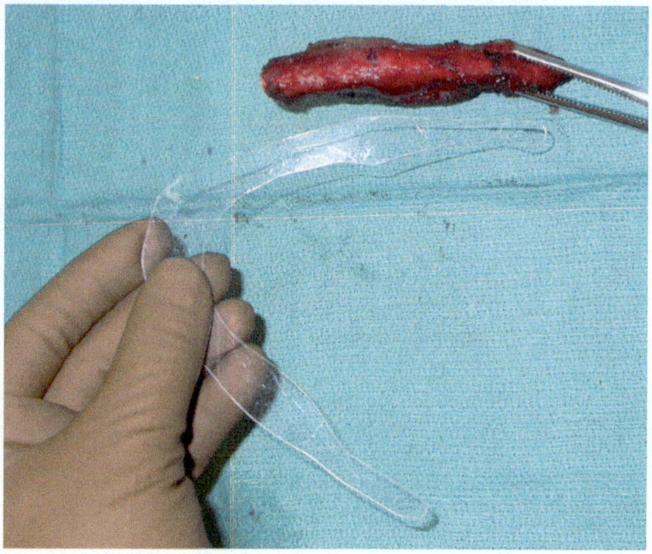

Fig. 14 Mandibular arch template utilized to determine angle of osteotomy in midbody of the neo-mandible

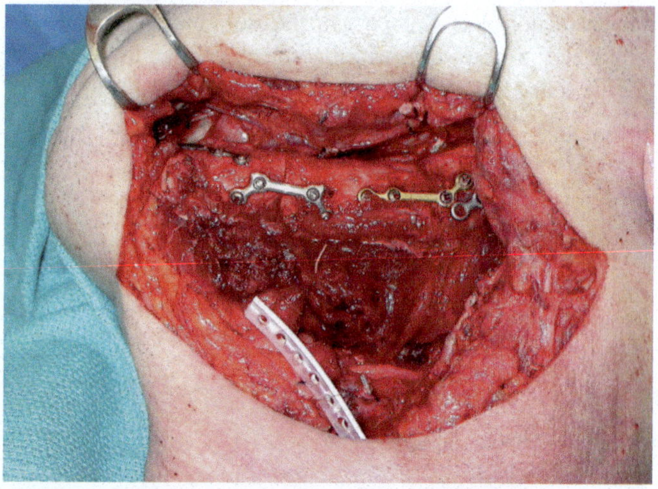

Fig. 16 Neo-mandible rigidly fixated to native mandible

If necessary, the condyle is autotransplanted onto the most proximal portion of the fibula to reconstruct the condyle (Fig. 15). The neo-mandible is rigidly fixed into the defect with miniplates once the flap pedicle is divided (Fig. 16).

The same approach can be used to reconstruct the maxillary segments. Usually, only a single template is necessary to reproduce the curvature of the maxilla.

Virtual Surgical Planning

The VSP process begins with the appropriate preoperative imaging. High-resolution CT scans of the mandible and fibula with 1 mm interval cuts are obtained and sent to a third-party vendor. A conference call is then arranged between the vendor and the oncologic and plastic surgeons. The vendor begins the process by demonstrating the mandible or maxilla on-screen, highlighting the location of tumor involvement. The ablative surgeon is then given control of the virtual scalpel to demonstrate the location of the osteotomies (Fig. 17). Next, the fibula is positioned on-screen to replace the removed areas of the mandible/maxilla (Fig. 18). The same location and number of osteotomies are performed as with the traditional templates described above. Once the virtual fibula reconstruction is complete (Fig. 19), dental implants can also be placed into the fibula. The location and depth of implant placement are determined at this time.

After completion of the conference call, acrylic cutting jigs for the tumor resection and the fibula are made through the process of additive printing. The products are fabricated and sent to the institution for preoperative sterilization.

In the operating room, the cutting jig(s) for the resection are placed on either the mandible or maxilla to facilitate mesial and distal bony cuts that include the tumor (Fig. 20). It is important that the cutting guides fit and adapt precisely to the intended location of the preoperative VSP. The best way to ensure appropriate positioning is for the vendor to design the guide around unique features of the bony anatomy, including curves and notches. For example, a guide that cups the mandibular angle has little chance for malposition, whereas a guide on the mid-body can easily slide mesially or distally. Perhaps the best method to ensure precise positioning is a guide based at the occlusion with an extension arm for the osteotomy. Once positioned, the guide is affixed to the bone with screws to void movement during the osteotomy. The entire osteotomy needs to be performed through the jig-cutting slot. Because the osteotomy plane is often angulated, not perpendicular to the buccal surface of the mandible, it is not sufficient to merely score the surface of the mandible with the saw.

A similar process is performed on the leg after the fibula is harvested (Fig. 21). While the peroneal vessel is still attached, the fibula cutting jig is adapted to the bone. Similar to mandible/maxilla jig placement, it is important that the fibula jig is positioned at the correct anatomic location, as designed during the VSP. The fibula shape can change quite significantly as it proceeds from proximal to distal; therefore, the guide will not adapt appropriately to the bone if positioned on the incorrect anatomic area. Once again, the jig is secured to the fibula with screws. If dental implants are intended, they are usually placed first, followed by osteotomies through the cutting slots. The most proximal and distal of the fibula osteotomies are complementary to those made by the ablative team. The jig is removed (Fig. 22), followed by rigid fixation using either miniplates or a reconstruction bar, depending upon surgeon preference. Custom-designed plates made through additive printing are used for maxillary reconstruction and delayed reconstruction or when immediate dental implants are placed (Fig. 23). The contoured fib-

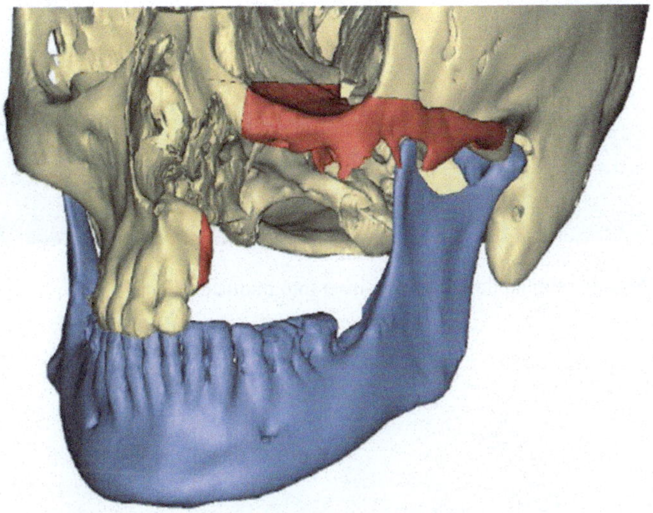

Fig. 17 Planned maxillary and zygoma resection in a patient with recurrent cancer who had a prior maxillectomy. Resection is highlighted in red

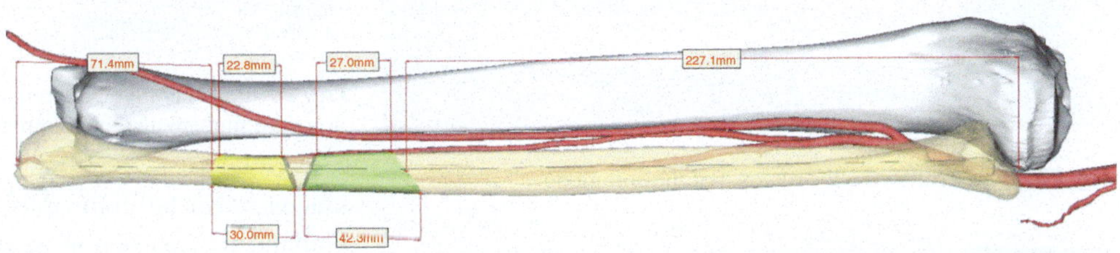

Fig. 18 Planned two-piece fibula flap reconstruction with a single closing wedge osteotomy

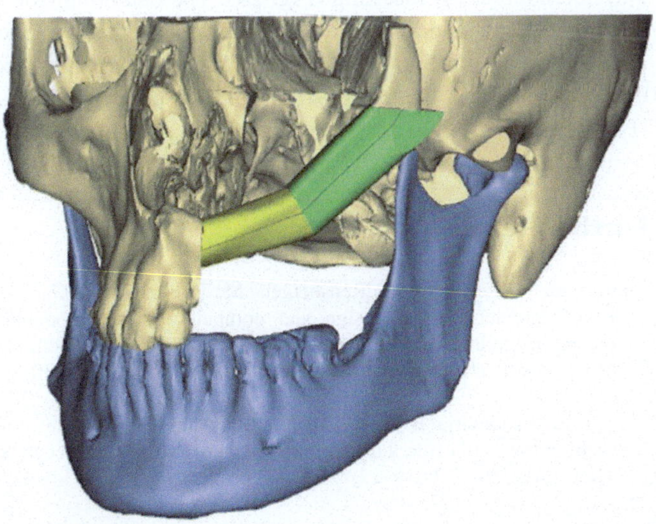

Fig. 19 Virtual reconstruction of the defect with the two-piece fibula flap

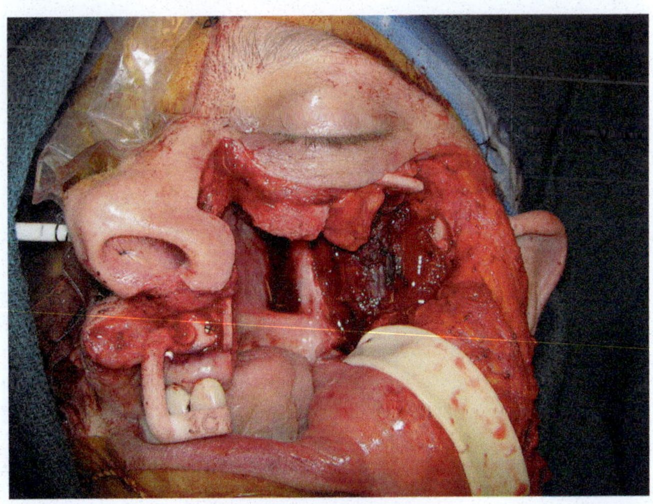

Fig. 20 Occlusal-based cutting jugs used to resect the remaining portions of the maxilla and zygoma

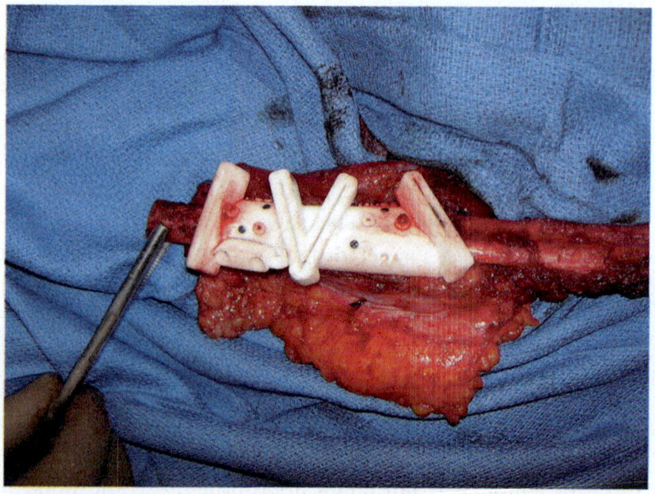

Fig. 21 Fibula cutting jig with slot for dental implants

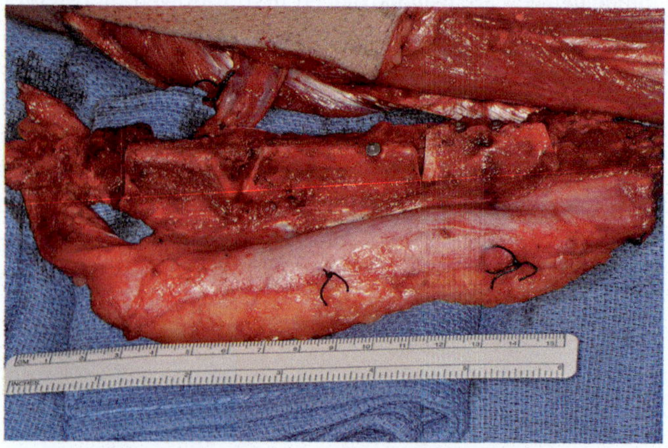

Fig. 22 Fibula following the removal of the cutting jig

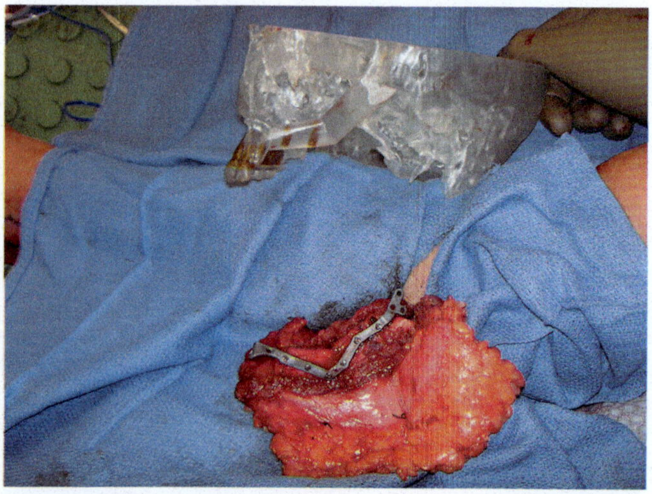

Fig. 23 Fibula plated with a prefabricated custom miniplate. The reconstruction is compared to a 3-D stereolithographic model

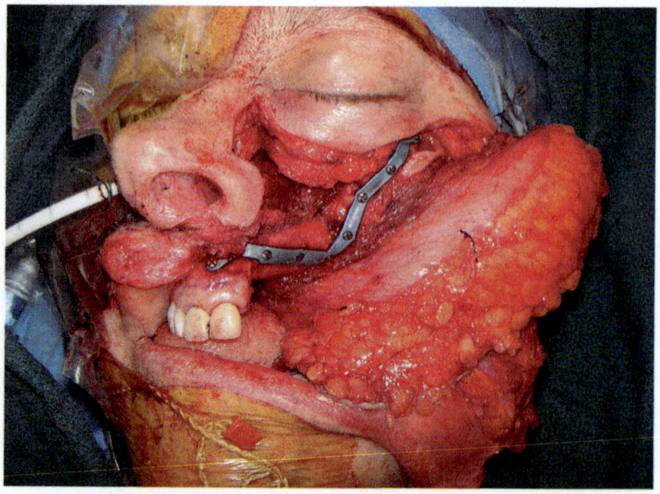

Fig. 24 Fibula flap following inset into midface defect

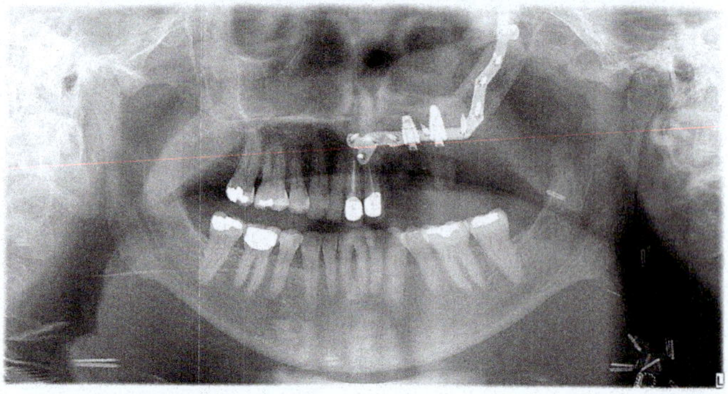

Fig. 25 Postoperative panoramic dental radiograph of the reconstruction with immediate dental implants

ula can also be compared to a 3-D acrylic model of the planned reconstruction to ensure accuracy with the virtual surgical plan (Fig. 23). The flap is brought up to the head and neck defect for insetting (Fig. 24). The osteotomies on the maxilla or mandible should be complementary to the ends of the fibula flap with perfect alignment. A Panorex demonstrates excellent apposition of the bone segments (Fig. 25).

Further Reading

Matros E, Albornoz CR, Rensberger M, Weimer K, Garfein ES. Computer-assisted design and computer-assisted modeling technique optimization and advantages over traditional methods of osseous flap reconstruction. J Reconstr Microsurg. 2014;30(5):289–96.

Matros E, Santamaria E, Cordeiro PG. Standardized templates for shaping the fibula free flap in mandible reconstruction. J Reconstr Microsurg. 2013;29:619–22.

Mandible: Lateral, Hemimandibular, Anterior

Luigi Chiarini, Alexandre Anesi, and Sara Negrello

We briefly describe the mandibular reconstructive principles related to specific defects, referring to the classification proposed by PG Cordeiro (see chapter "Classification System for Mandibulectomy Defects") [1].

Type I Defects

The importance of the anterior mandible for maintaining projection and support of the lower face and the potential for dental implant osseointegration makes bony reconstruction the dominant consideration in type I (anterior) defects (Figs. 1–3). Type I defects involve through and through the anterior arch, including the symphysis, but may also include one or both parasymphyses, e.g. the canine tooth-bearing bone.

Type IA is appropriately reconstructed with an osseous (bone only) fibula.

Type IB and IC defects can be reconstructed with an osteocutaneous fibula flap, with the skin island used for intraoral lining (in type IB defects) or skin replacement (type IC) (Figs. 4 and 5). Type ID defects require abundant soft tissue restoration of both intraoral structures and skin. In some cases, a single fibula skin island can be folded with a strip of skin deepithelialized, to go through a tunnel from oral to external areas; this technique is suitable if the intraoral includes the lower buccoalveolar sulci (vestibule of mouth) or the lower alveolus and gingiva (lower gum). Double skin paddle fibula flap can be performed safely if two perforators are identified: two distinct skin islands can be positioned with greater ease. Alternatively, a separate radial forearm fasciocutaneous flap can be used (one used for intraoral lining and one for skin) [1, 4].

L. Chiarini (✉) · A. Anesi · S. Negrello
Cranio-Maxillo-Facial Surgery Unit, University Hospital of Modena, Modena, Italy
e-mail: luigi.chiarini@unimore.it; alexandre.anesi@unimore.it

To completely restore the anterior mandible, it is necessary to overcome the limited height of the fibula compared to the native symphyseal and parasymphyseal region; adequate bone height is a precondition for dental implants planning (see chapter "Bone Augmentation") [5].

In fibular modelling, particular attention is given to maintaining good vascularity of the bone segments by minimizing the number of osteotomies, although blood perfusion was ensured by intact periosteal circulation. It has been shown that it is possible to perform multiple osteotomies (of as little as 1 cm) without compromising the viability of the bone blocks [6]. In short people and small mandible when the distal mandibular osteotomic line is just anterior to the molar region because of resection planning, the distal fibular block is consequently short and has uncertain vascularization. In our clinical practice, fibula segments shorter than 2 cm are endangered for insufficient blood flow.

Type II Defects

Type II (hemimandible) (Fig. 6) defects comprehend the entire hemimandible from the parasymphysis to the ipsilateral ascending ramus and sometimes include the condyle. The degree of bony deficit is important; therefore, the fibula is indicated in most instances because of the bone's high quality and quantity. As an increasing magnitude of posterior soft tissue is resected, however, closure of the soft tissue defect and restoration of the intraoral surfaces take priority. For aesthetic restoration, it is conceptually ideal to replace the entire bony deficit to maintain the shape and contours of the lateral aspect of the lower face. In terms of function, there is minimal deficit if the anterior arch and contralateral hemimandible remain intact.

When the condyle cannot be preserved, prosthetic replacement in the temporomandibular joint is not ideal treatment owing to the risk of material failure or erosion of the temporal bone over the years, especially in young patients [8, 9].

G. De Santis et al. (eds.), *Atlas of Mandibular and Maxillary Reconstruction with the Fibula Flap*,
https://doi.org/10.1007/978-3-030-10684-3_5

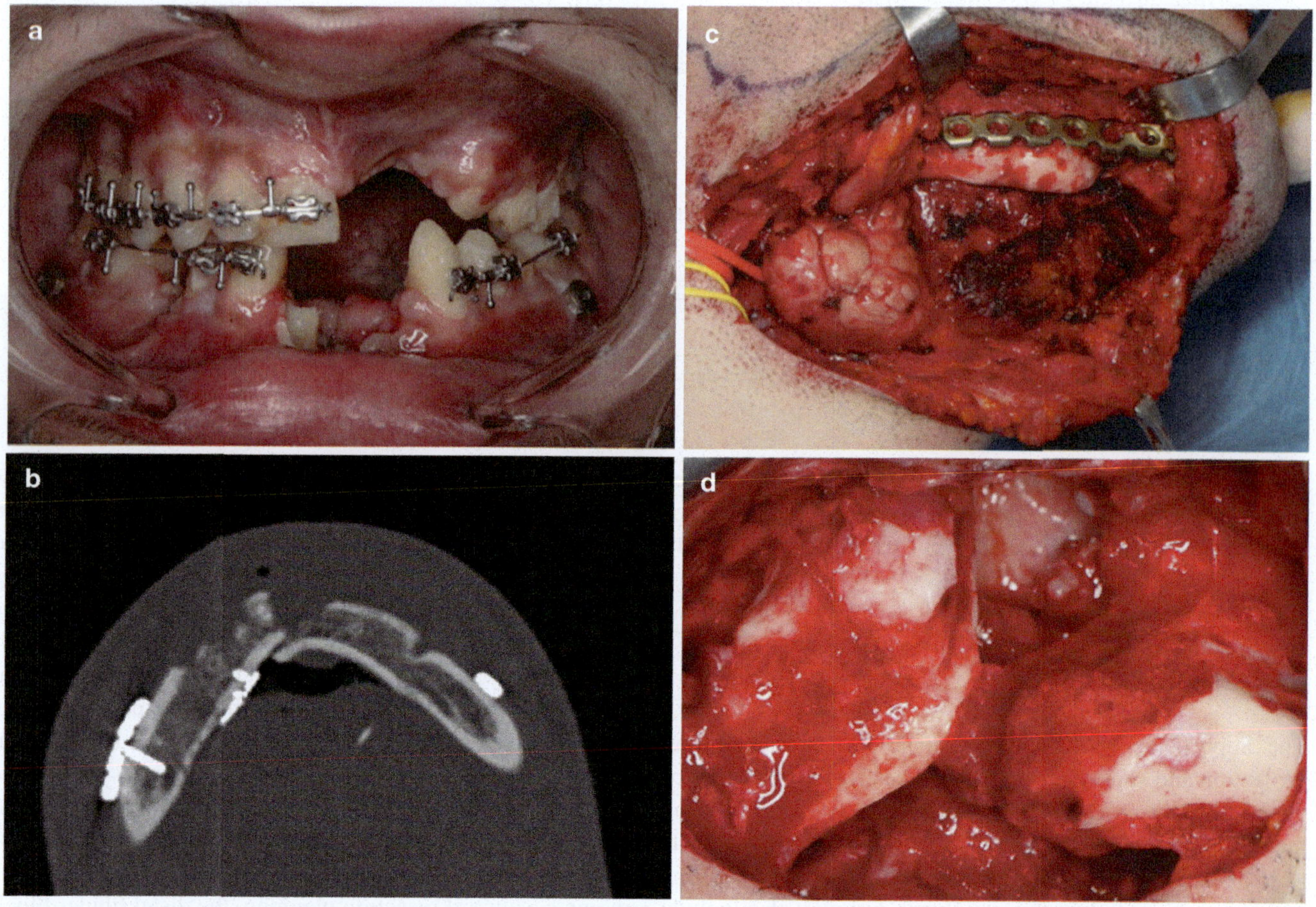

Fig. 1 (**a** and **b**) Symphyseal and parasymphyseal defect due to a non-union after a significant blunt trauma, resulting in a type IA defect (according to PG Cordeiro's classification). (**c**) Reconstruction plate for transient fixation of mandibular stumps. (**d**) Segmental mandibular defect after plate removal

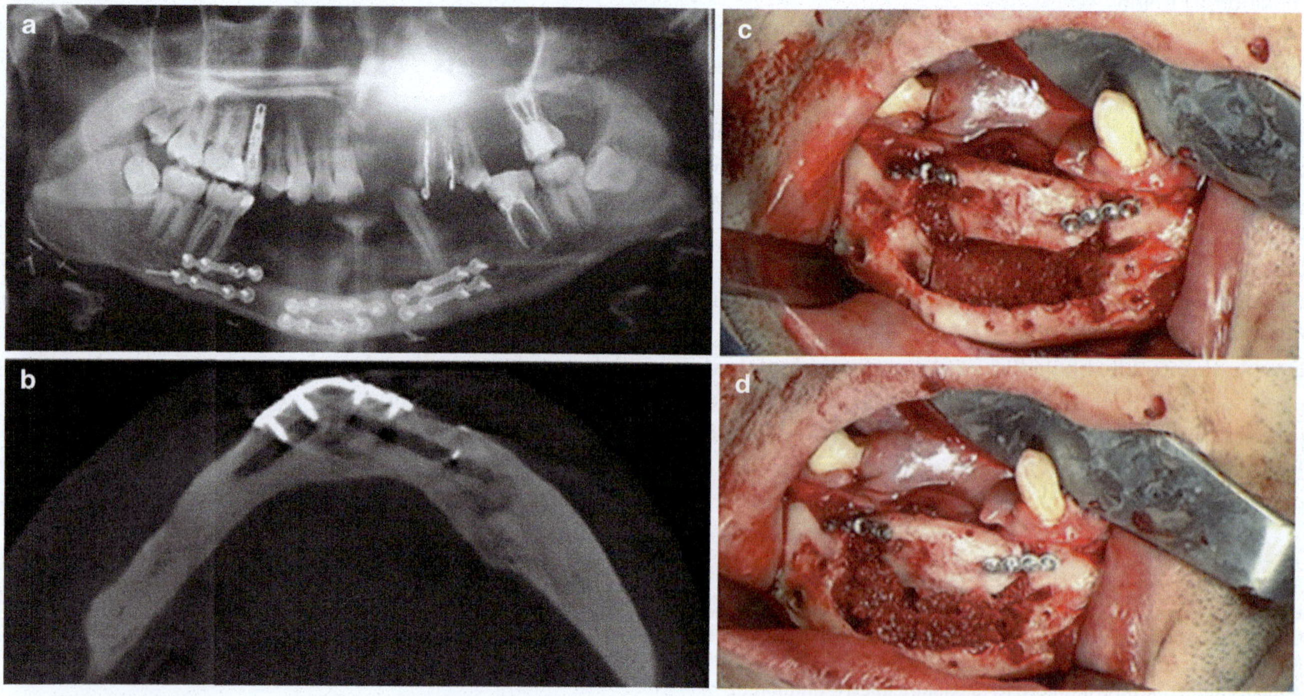

Fig. 2 (**a**) Postoperative orthopantomograph of two-fibula segment reconstruction. (**b**) Postoperative axial cone beam CT scan with satisfactory bone union. The vertical symphyseal discrepancy is high. (**c**) Fibula split was performed by a piezosurgical osteotome. (**d**) Cancellous iliac crest autologous bone was utilized for inlay graft [2, 3]

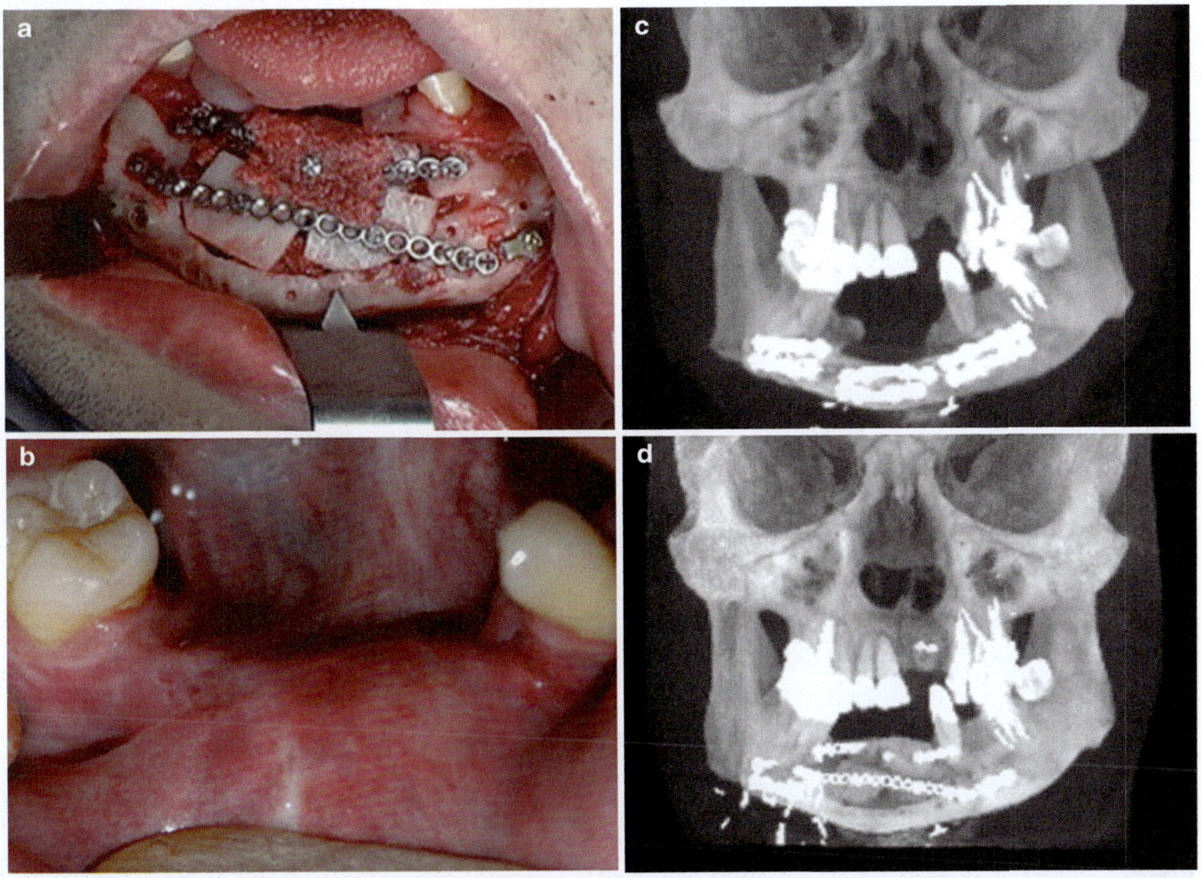

Fig. 3 (**a**) Corticocancellous iliac graft is applied at the vestibular surface of the neosymphysis to complete the vertical restoration of the mandible. (**b**) Oral appearance with complete mucosal healing. (**c** and **d**) Comparison between preoperative and postoperative coronal view by cone beam CT with reconstruction of adequate vertical dimension in symphyseal and parasymphyseal areas

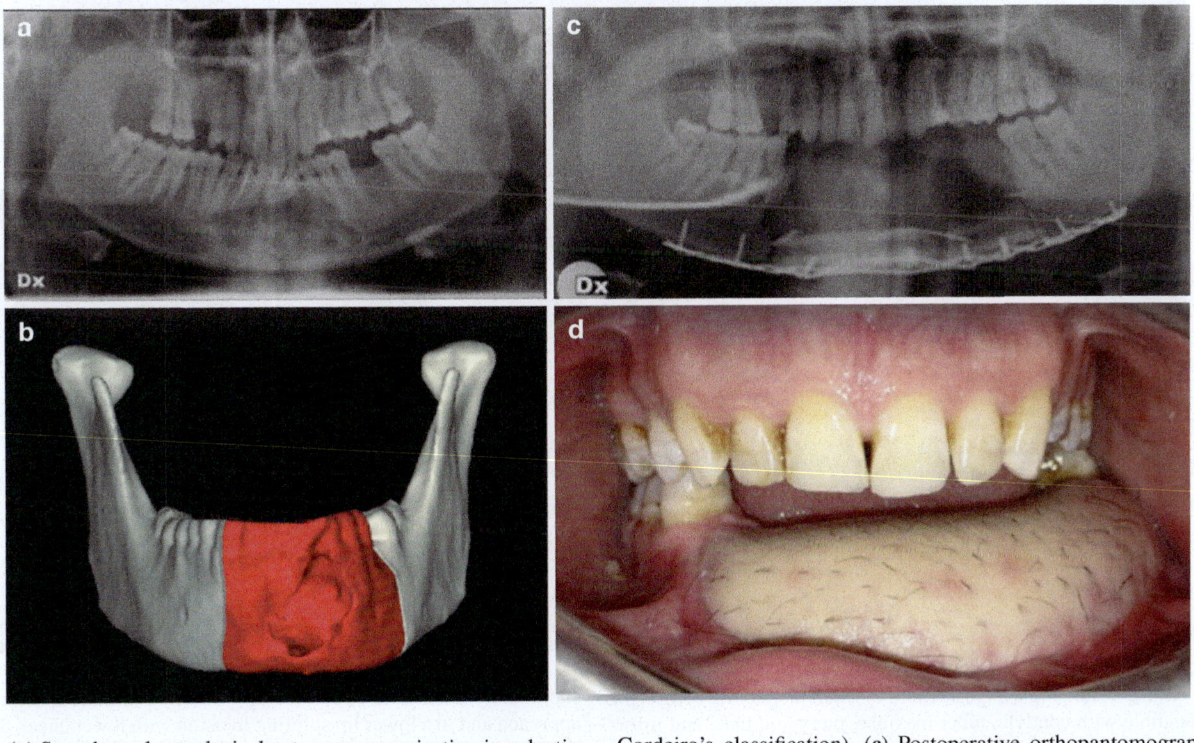

Fig. 4 (**a**) Symphyseal osteolysis due to rare cancerization in a dentigerous cyst (note the 33 tooth impacted). (**b**) Digital planning of the resection, which corresponds to a type IB defect (according to PG Cordeiro's classification). (**c**) Postoperative orthopantomograph with the two-fibula segment reconstruction. (**d**) Postoperative intraoral view with the intraoral skin paddle

Fig. 5 Preoperative and postoperative frontal view of the young patient of Fig. 4

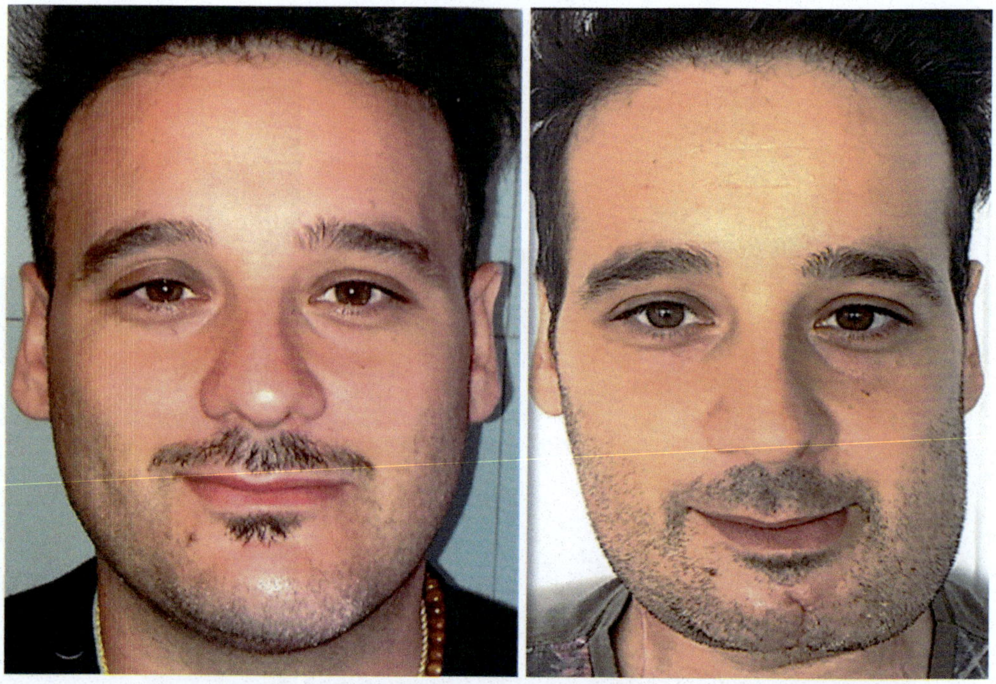

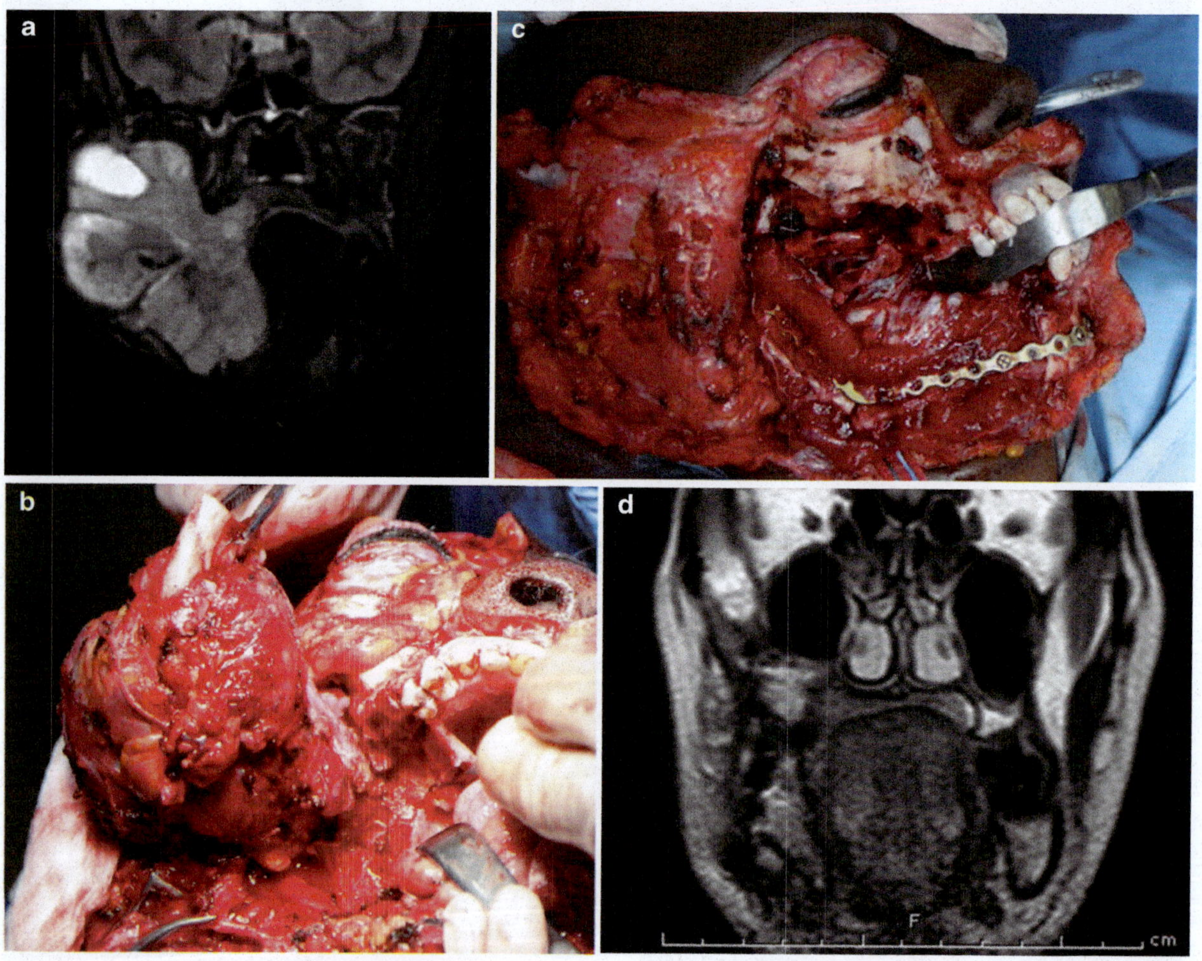

Fig. 6 (**a**) MRI showing a huge adenoid cyst carcinoma involving right hemimandible with condyle, tuber maxillae, pterygoid plate and infratemporal fossa. (**b**) Type IIB2 defect (according to PG Cordeiro's classification) is given after hemimandibulectomy with the condyle by means of Shah's approach (Weber-Fergusson incision – subciliary + supraciliary extension, continued upwards in a unilateral hemicoronal approach and in a lower lip splitting incision with lower cheek flap) [7]. (**c**) Right ramus and mandible body reconstruction with fibula flap (no skin paddle is needed). (**d**) Postoperative MRI

Fibula ramus reconstruction placed in the glenoid fossa is possible: proximal extremity of fibula rounds up due to the function against the temporomandibular disc. In these patients, oral function is preserved without ankylosis [10]. Maintaining the fibula in the glenoid fossa can be a surgical challenge. The use of intermaxillary fixation allows the fibula to be applied directly to the temporomandibular disc in the glenoid fossa and establish the proper posterior facial height. Wire fixation of the fibular extremities to articular eminence or to postglenoid process is possible. However, direct suspension of the flap in the fossa with sutures or wire is difficult and imprecise [11, 12].

Nevertheless, translation movement of a neocondyle will not be possible, with consequent asymmetry in opening and in protrusive movements of the mandible [13].

Masseter muscle deficiency occurs in composite resection of mandibular ramus and angle. The hypotrophic masseter region is aesthetically impaired and can be restored by fillers or, better yet, through lipofilling [14].

The proper orientation and angulation of the ramus-and-condyle segment of the fibula before fixation is more accurate and simpler if a preoperative CAD/CAM plan is performed [15].

Type IIA defects are best reconstructed with an osseous fibula flap.

Type IIB 1 defects necessitate intraoral tissue reconstruction and a myofascial lining, which can also be performed with myofascial fibula flap (with parts of either peroneus longus or soleus or flexor hallucis longus muscles). The bulking effect of a skin island near the oropharynx is thus avoided [16].

Type IIB2 defects need large soft tissue volume for intraoral resurfacing and to avoid orocutaneous fistula in the neck. Myofascial or osteocutaneous fibula flap rarely manages to provide enough tissue. A revascularized soft tissue flap, such as the vertical rectus abdominis myocutaneous flap, provides wide skin surface, muscle and adipose tissue volume (Figs. 6–8). This flap does not have any osseous component and can be associated with fibula flap [17].

Type IIC defects are characterized by extensive bony requirements and skin resection. Fibula osteocutaneous flap is suitable for reconstruction of these defects with similar tissues.

Type IID defects are due to large composite resection. The combined procedure which includes resection of a portion of the mandible in continuity with the neck dissection and resection of the primary intraoral lesion has come to be known as the "commando procedure" or the "composite resection" [18].

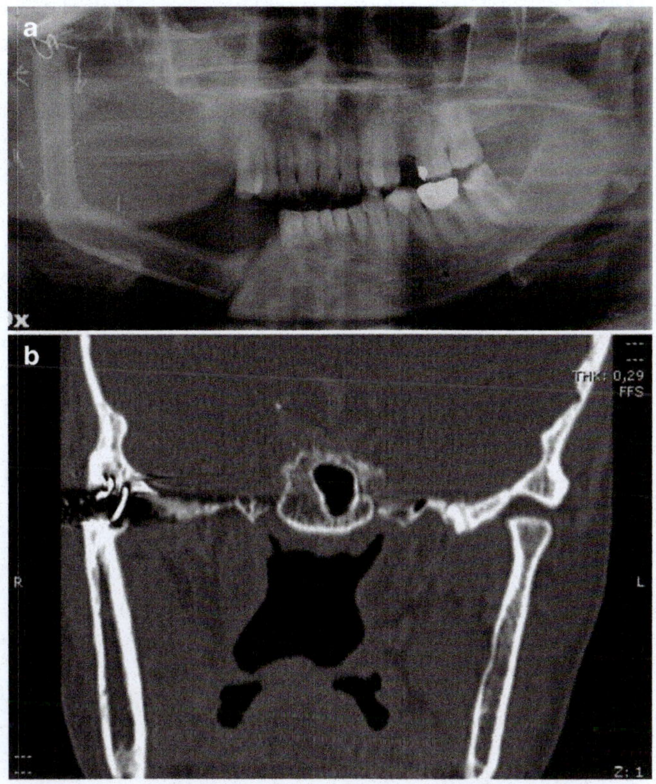

Fig. 7 (**a**) Postoperative orthopantomograph after plate removal. (**b**) CT scan shows wire fixation of fibula extremity in the right glenoid fossa

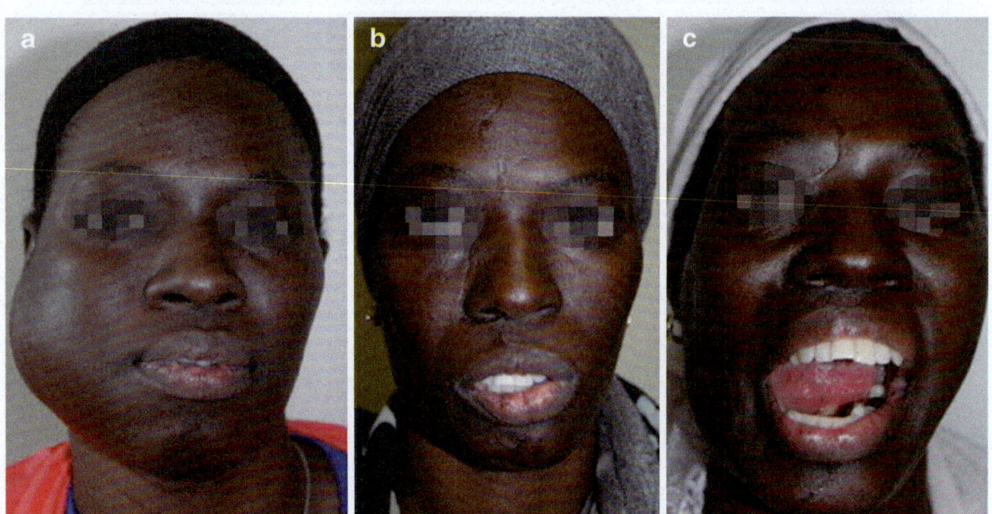

Fig. 8 Preoperative (**a**) and postoperative (**b** and **c**) frontal view of the patient of Figs. 6 and 7. No right facial nerve deficit

Advanced oncologic disease of these patients needs fast and effective healing to access adjuvant treatments [19]. For this reason, large soft tissue free flaps are preferred, such as two-skin-island vertical rectus abdominis myocutaneous flap or latissimus dorsi flap. Fibula osteocutaneous flap plus a radial forearm flap is also described by many authors [1, 4, 17, 20].

Type III Defects

Finally, type III defects have lack of bony tissue in the lateral body/angle of the mandible. The fibula osseous flap is best for reconstructing a type IIIA defect. Type IIIB defects, intraoral lining defects, are best reconstructed with the fibula osteocutaneous flap (Figs. 9–11). When tumours involve the ascending ramus, the main defect is the surface area of the lateral oropharyngeal mucosa, while the teeth-bearing retromolar area has limited functional consequence. For this defect, a radial forearm fasciocutaneous flap is suitable because it provides thin and pliable skin; for bone reconstruction, a radial forearm osteocutaneous flap is also described [20, 21].

Type IIIC defects can derive from skin or parotid gland tumours. Compared to wide skin defects, bony functional consequences of resection are minimal; vertical

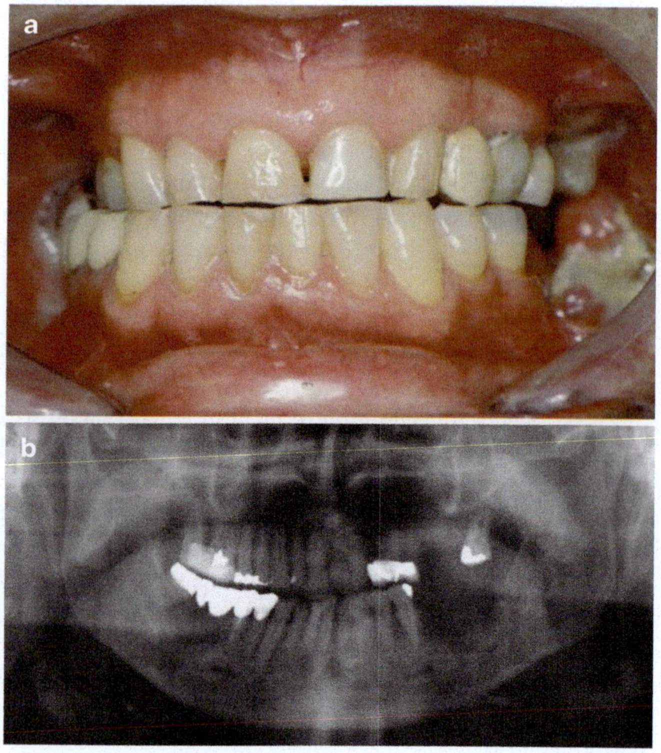

Fig. 9 Bilateral osteoradionecrosis of the mandibular body. (**a**) Left oral exposed and necrotic bone. (**b**) In orthopantomograph osteolysis is more evident on left mandibular side

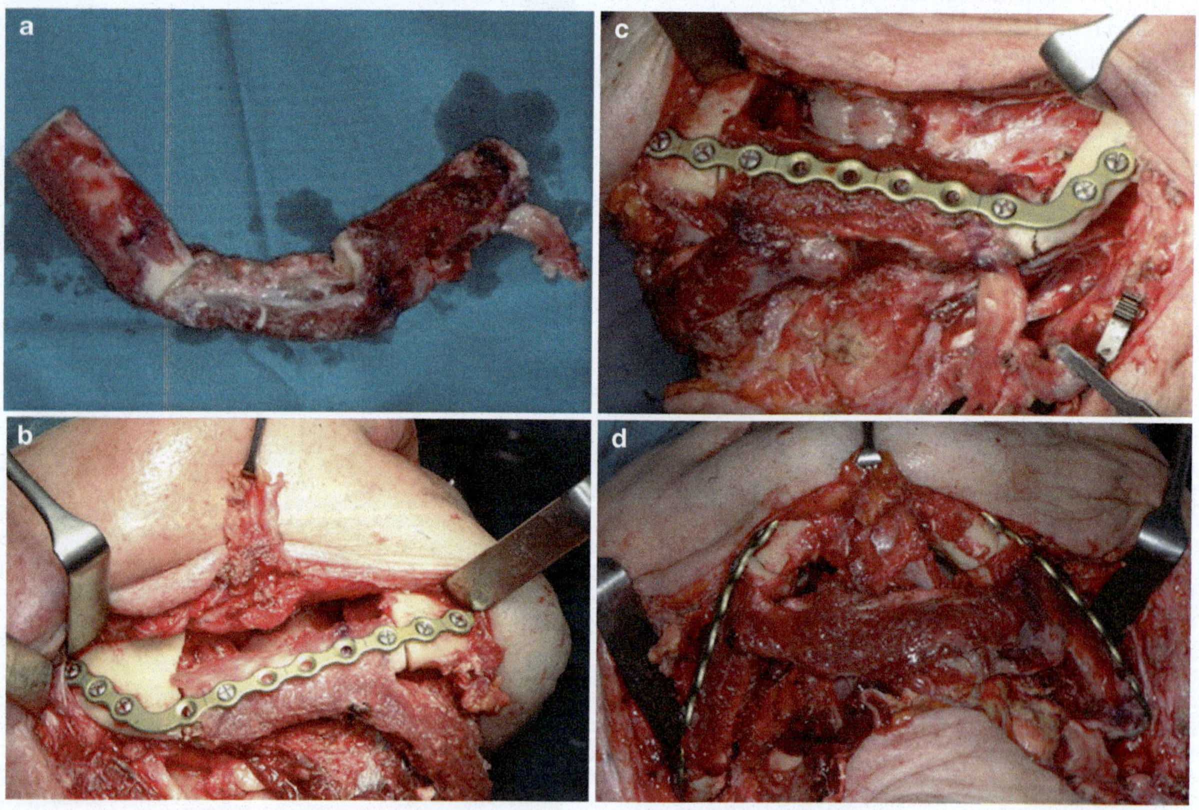

Fig. 10 (**a**) Bilateral mandibular body resection was performed, preserving symphyseal and parasymphyseal region. The resection volume corresponds to bilateral type IIIB defect (according to PG Cordeiro's classification). A unique fibula flap reconstructed bilateral mandibular body by means of a large segment was removed from the medial third of the fibula, leaving the periosteal layer intact. (**b**) Right mandibular reconstruction with the fibula flap, fixed with a reconstruction plate. (**c**) Left mandibular reconstruction with the fibula flap. (**d**) Vision from the bottom of the completed reconstruction with the vascular pedicle of the flap passing in submental area

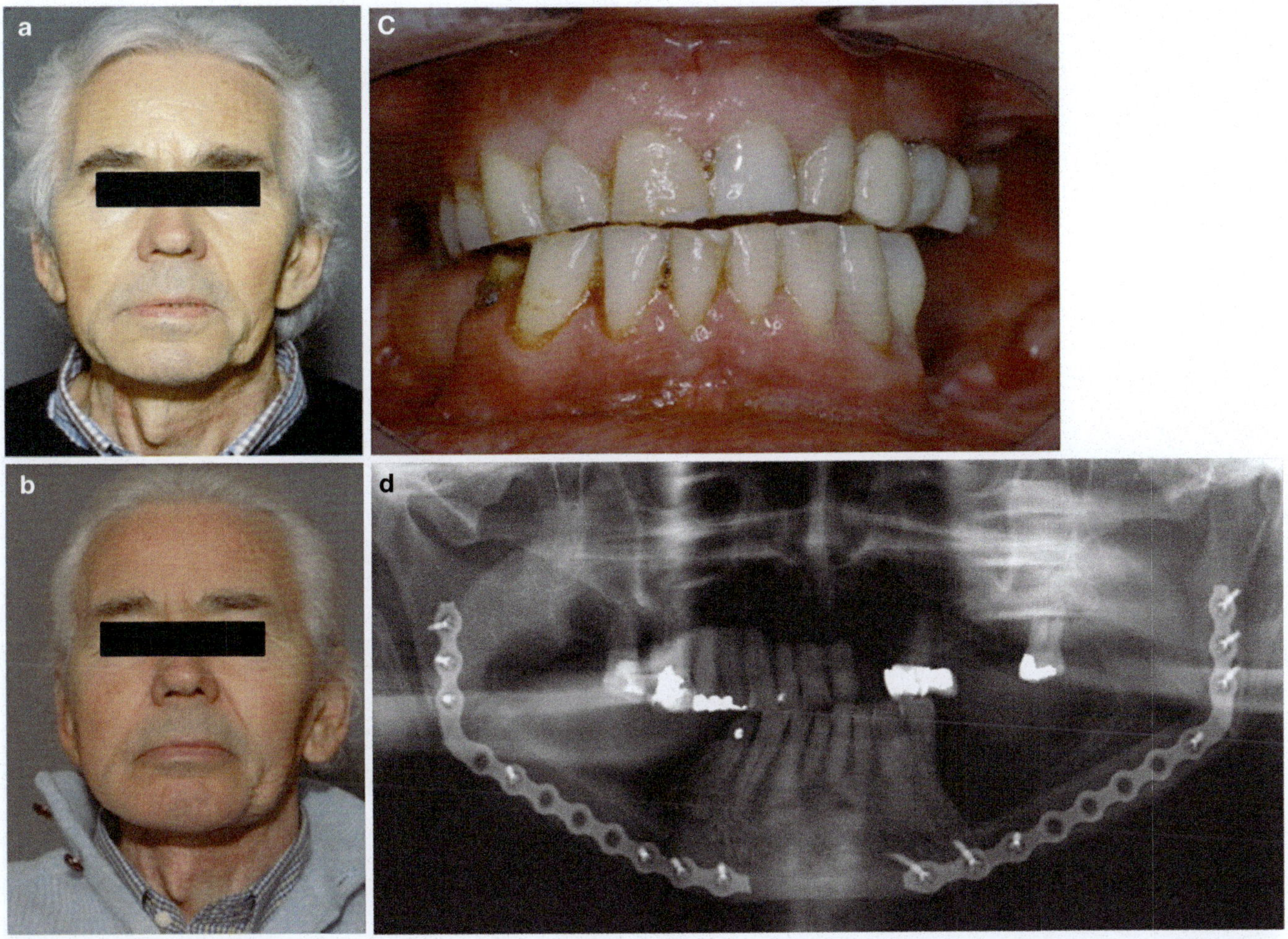

Fig. 11 (**a** and **b**) Preoperative and postoperative frontal view of the patient. (**c**) Dental occlusion was preserved. (**d**) postoperative orthopantomograph

rectus abdominis myocutaneous flap, anterolateral thigh flap or latissimus dorsi flap are appropriate. The scapula osteocutaneous flap provides well-matched skin resurfacing and a modest amount of bone adequate for the defect [22].

Type IIID defects are usually created after resection of locally advanced tumours originating in the gingiva or cheek mucosa, which extend inwards to the floor of the mouth and tongue and outwards into the mandible and skin. A fibula osteocutaneous flap with a large, folded skin island or multiple skin islands is needed. For the largest defects, a double flap (fibula osteocutaneous flap externally, radial forearm fasciocutaneous or vertical rectus abdominis myocutaneous intraorally) may be required [1] (Figs. 12–16).

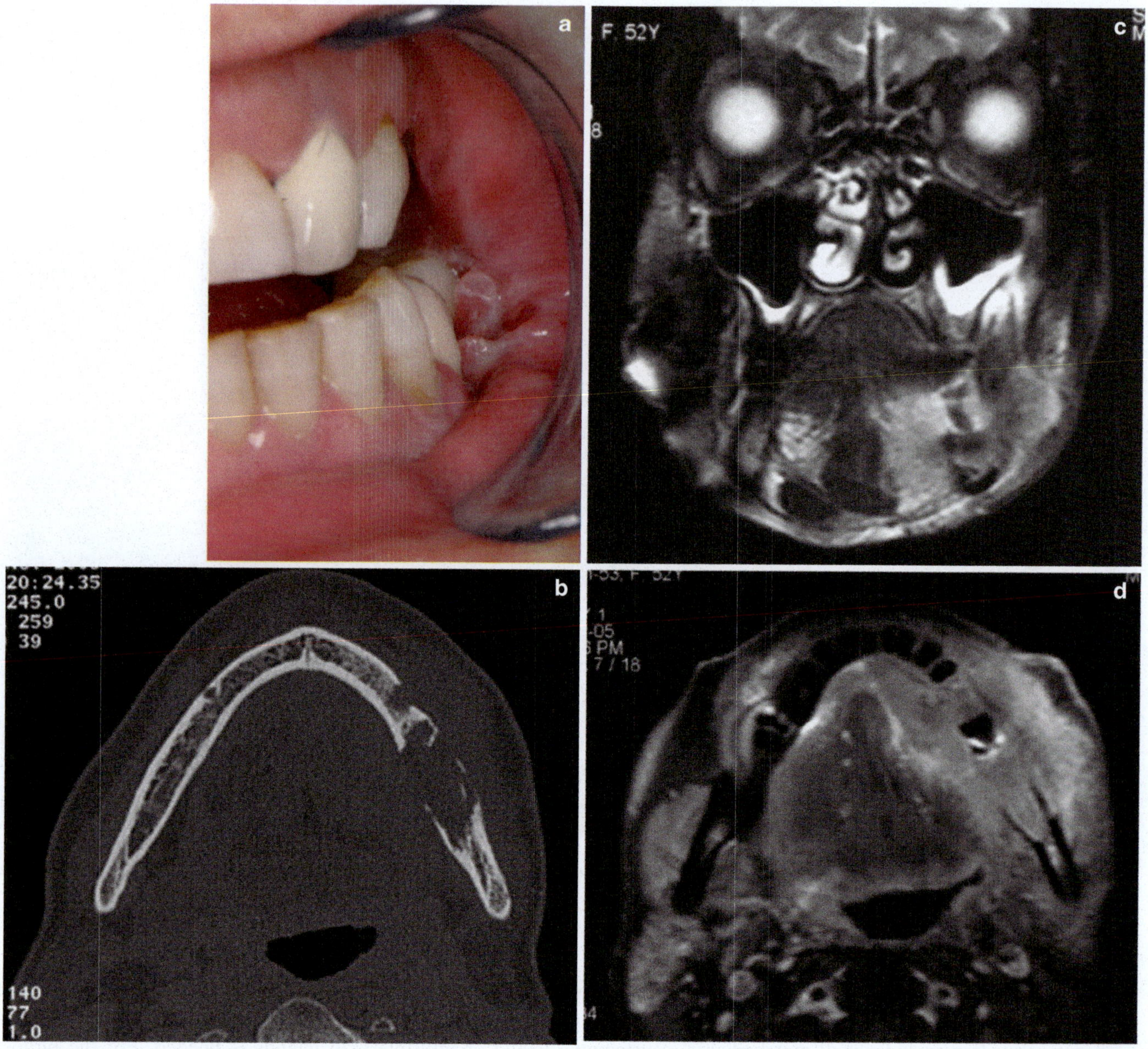

Fig. 12 (**a**) Extensive oral cancer relapse from lower alveolus and gingiva, afterwards a previous surgical and adjuvant radiotherapy treatment performed in another hospital. (**b**) CT scan shows the lateral left mandible (body, angle) infiltration. (**c** and **d**) Coronal and axial MRI: floor of the mouth, the tongue, the cheek skin, the upper alveolus and the hypopharynx are involved

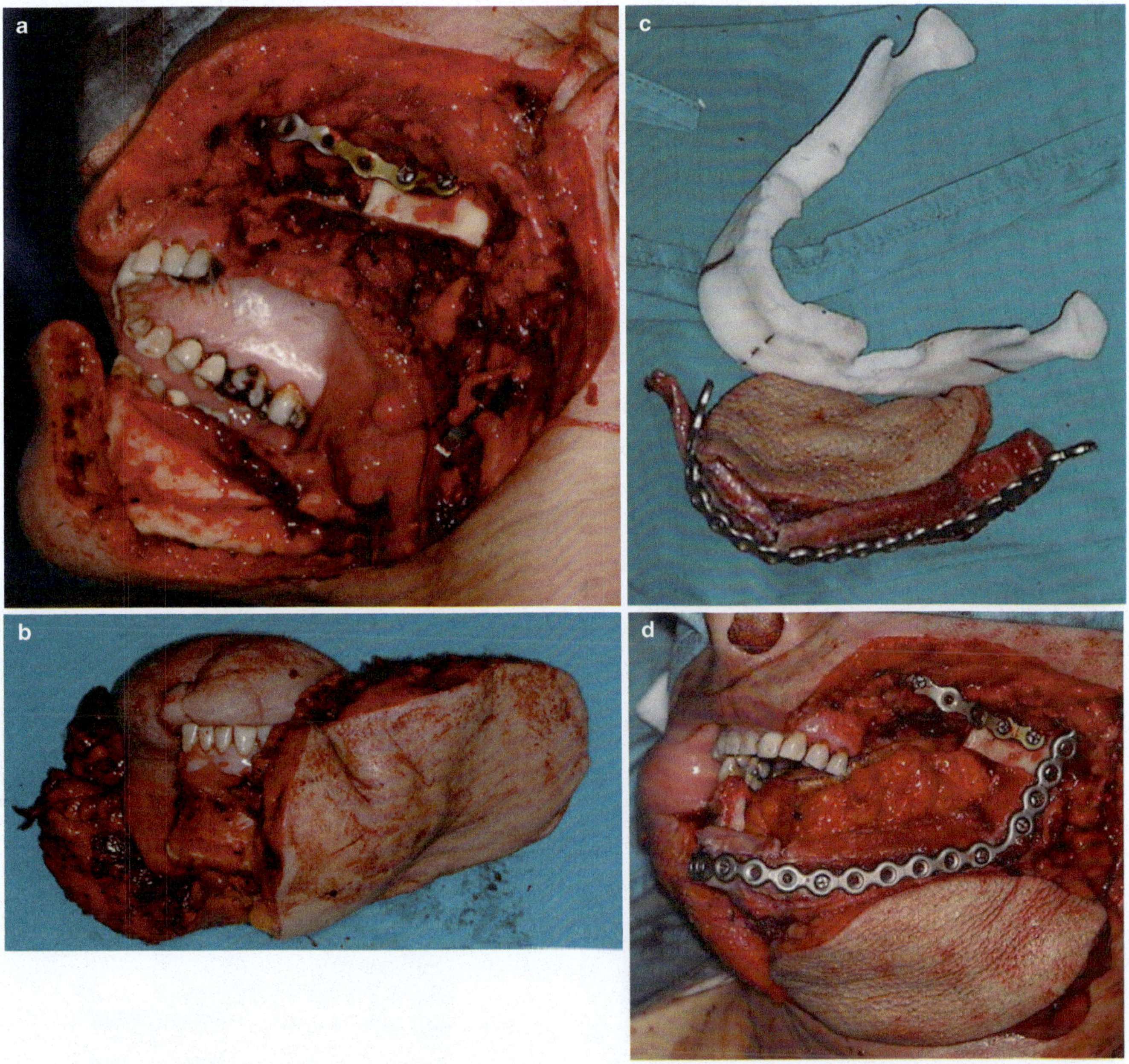

Fig. 13 (**a**) A composite resection was performed ("commando operation"): the left lateral mandible, the whole tongue and the floor of the mouth, the left upper alveolus and the larynx were resected. (**b**) The surgical specimen obtained with an en bloc resection. (**c**) The fibula flap shaping according to the stereolithographic model. (**d**) A transverse rectus abdominis muscle flap has already been positioned for the tongue when the fibula is fixed with a reconstruction plate (2.7 mm); the fibula skin island is used to replace the laterocervical skin. The resection volume corresponds to a type IIID defect (according to PG Cordeiro's classification)

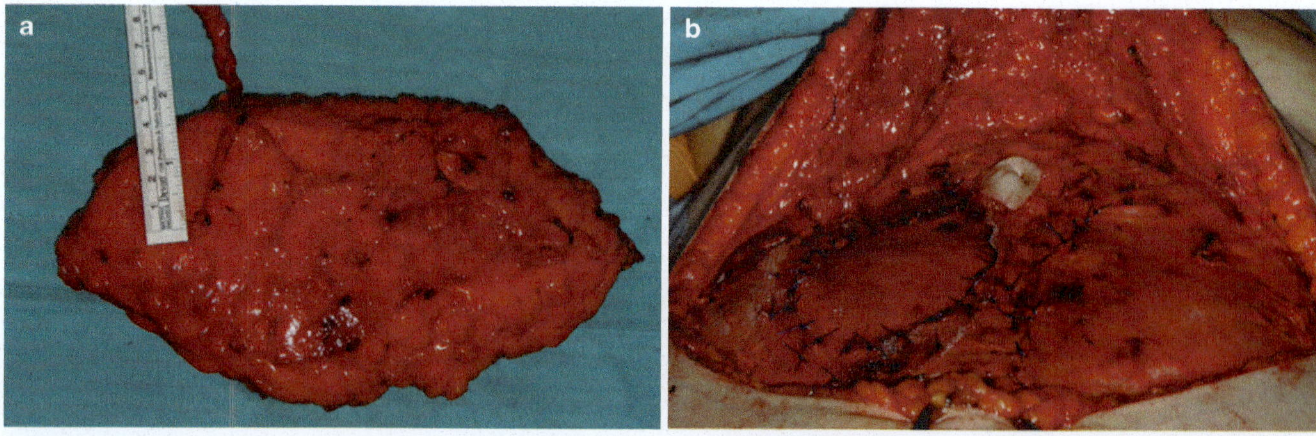

Fig. 14 The extensive skin resection of the cheek required deep inferior epigastric artery perforator flap. (**a**) The flap has already been harvested. (**b**) The abdominoplasty was ready, and the onlay Prolene mesh was sutured for restoration of the abdominal wall fascia, whereas the transverse rectus abdominis muscle flap has been already raised

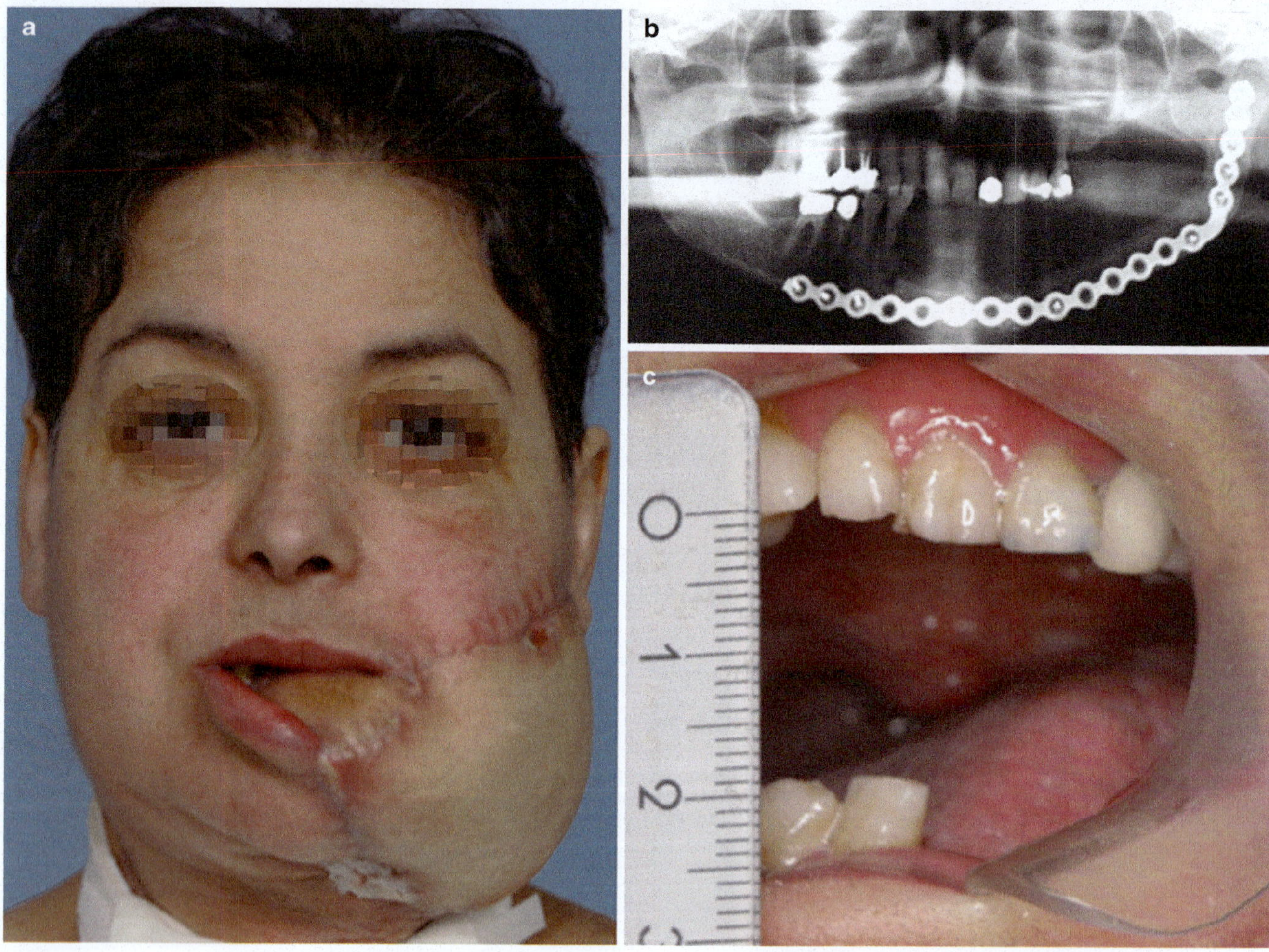

Fig. 15 (**a**) Short-term postoperative frontal view with labial incompetence and cheek bulk. (**b**) Postoperative orthopantomograph. (**c**) Sufficient mouth opening, considering the significant fibrosis related to previous radiation therapy

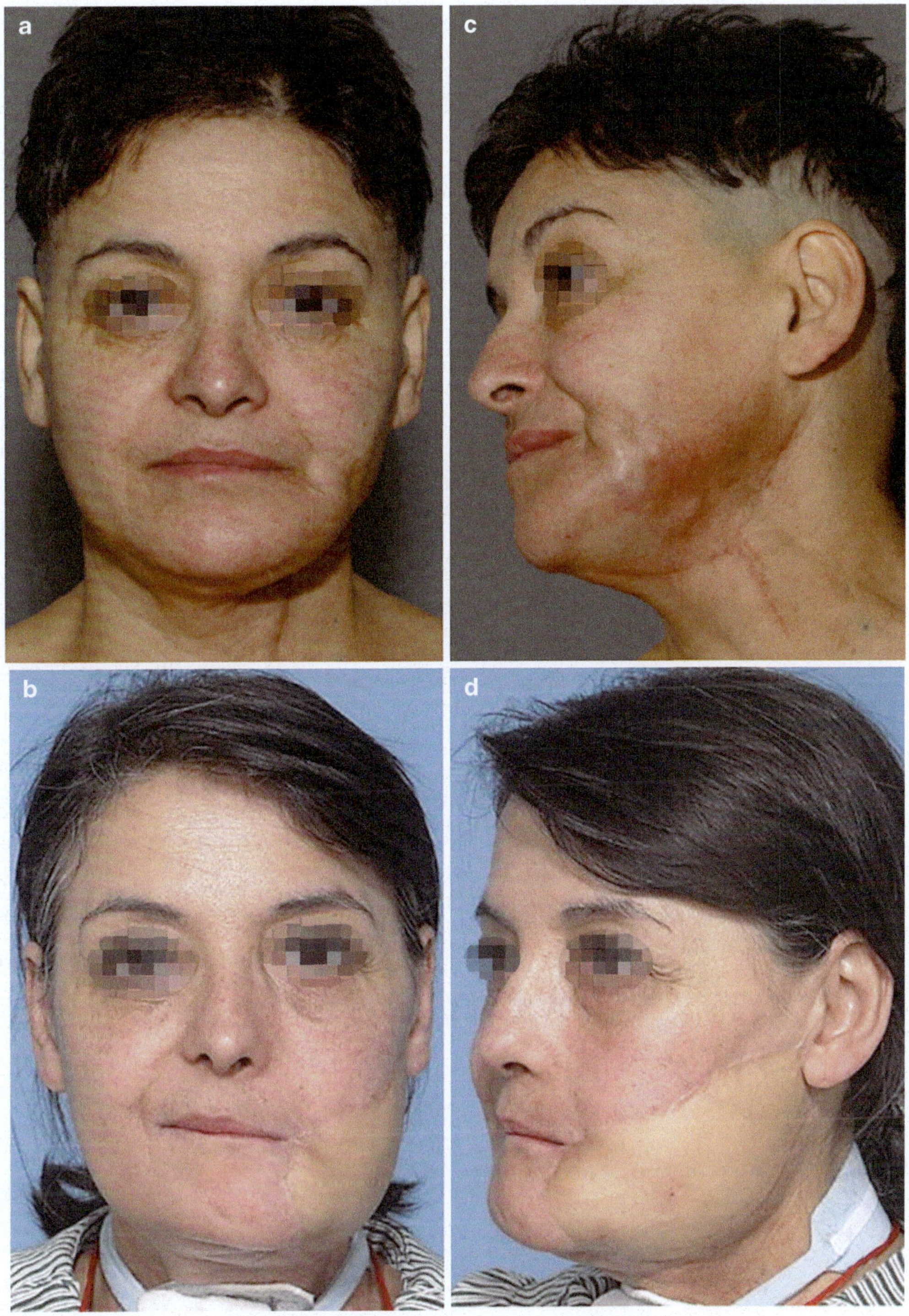

Fig. 16 Frontal and lateral views of the patient in Fig. 9, (**a** and **c**) preoperative and postoperative (**b** and **d**) (5 years after surgery). A defatting of cervical skin paddle and a left oral commissure reconstruction were performed

References

1. Cordeiro PG, Henderson PW, Matros E. A 20-year experience with 202 segmental mandibulectomy defects: a defect classification system, algorithm for flap selection, and surgical outcomes. Plast Reconstr Surg. 2018;141(4):571e–81e.
2. Anesi A, Ferretti M, Cavani F, Salvatori R, Bianchi M, Russo A, Chiarini L, Palumbo C. Structural and ultrastructural analyses of bone regeneration in rabbit cranial osteotomy: Piezosurgery versus traditional osteotomes. J Craniomaxillofac Surg. 2018;46(1):107–18. https://doi.org/10.1016/j.jcms.2017.10.004. Epub 2017 Oct 12
3. Turra M, Bertossi D, Bissolotti G, Anesi A, Chiarini L, Nocini PF. O.095 Genioplasty with piezosurgery. J Craniofac Surg. 2008;36(Suppl 1):S24. https://doi.org/10.1016/S1010-5182(08)71219-8.
4. Jones NF, Vögelin E, Markowitz BL, Watson JP. Reconstruction of composite through-and-through mandibular defects with a double skin paddle fibular osteocutaneous flap. Plast Reconstr Surg. 2003;112:758–65.
5. Bedogni A, Anesi A, Fior A, Bettini G, Nocini PF. Microsurgical reconstruction of the mandible in a patient with evans syndrome: a case report and review of the literature. J Reconstr Microsurg. 2013;29(8):545–50. https://doi.org/10.1055/s-0033-1348898. Epub 2013 Jun 26. Review
6. Bähr W. Blood supply of small fibula segments: an experimental study on human cadavers. J Craniomaxillofac Surg. 1998;26(3):148–52.
7. Salgarelli AC, Bellini P, Magnoni C, Anesi A, Collini M. Synergistic use of local flaps for total lower lip reconstruction. Dermatol Surg. 2011;37(11):1666–70. https://doi.org/10.1111/j.1524-4725.2011.02151.x. Epub 2011 Sep 14
8. Gilliot B, Siefert J, Caillot A, Soubeyrand E, Compère JF, Bénateau H. Condylar remodeling after temporomandibular joint reconstruction with fibula free flap. Rev Stomatol Chir Maxillofac Chir Orale. 2015;116:72–6.
9. Chiarini L, Figurelli S, Ghidini A, Nocini PF, Procacci P, Rubini C, Lo Muzio L, Lo Russo L. An unusual case of giant cell tumour involving the middle cranial fossa, originating from soft tissues of the temporomandibular joint. Acta Neurochir. 2009;151(12):1685–7. https://doi.org/10.1007/s00701-009-0296-3. Epub 2009 Apr 3
10. Guyot L, Oliver R, Layoun W, Cheynet F, Bellot-Samson V, Chossegros C, et al. Long-term radiologic findings following reconstruction of the condyle with fibular free flaps. J Craniomaxillofac Surg. 2004;32:98–102.
11. Engroff SL. Fibula flap reconstruction of the condyle in disarticulation resections of the mandible: a case report and review of the technique. Oral Surg Oral Med Oral Pathol Oral Radiol Endod. 2005;100:661–5.
12. Hidalgo DA. Condyle transplantation in free flap mandible reconstruction. Plast Reconstr Surg. 1994;93:770–81.
13. Chiarini L, Albanese M, Anesi A, Galzignato PF, Mortellaro C, Nocini P, Bertossi D. Surgical treatment of unilateral condylar hyperplasia with piezosurgery. J Craniofac Surg. 2014;25(3):808–10. https://doi.org/10.1097/SCS.0000000000000699.
14. Salgarelli AC, Anesi A, Bellini P, Pollastri G, Tanza D, Barberini S, Chiarini L. How to improve retromandibular transmasseteric anteroparotid approach for mandibular condylar fractures: our clinical experience. Int J Oral Maxillofac Surg. 2013;42(4):464–9. https://doi.org/10.1016/j.ijom.2012.12.012.. Epub 2013 Feb 8
15. Bao T, He J, Yu C, Zhao W, Lin Y, Wang H, et al. Utilization of a prebent plate-positioning surgical guide system in precise mandibular reconstruction with a free fibula flap. Oral Oncol. 2017;75:133–9.
16. Fan S, Wang YY, Wu DH, Lai DL, Feng YH, Yu X, et al. Intraoral lining with the fibular osteomyofascial flap without a skin paddle during maxillary and mandibular reconstruction. Head Neck. 2016;38(Suppl 1):E832–6.
17. Wei FC, Demirkan F, Chen HC, Chen IH. Double free flaps in reconstruction of extensive composite mandibular defects in head and neck cancer. Plast Reconstr Surg. 1999;103(1):39–47.
18. Martin HE. Surgery of head and neck tumors. New York: Paul B. Hoeber, Inc., Medical Bk. Dept. of Harper & Bros.; 1957.
19. Marella GL, Raschellà F, Solinas M, Mutolo P, Potenza S, Milano F, Mauriello S, Caggiano B, Rondinelli P, Anesi A, Migaldi M. The diagnostic delay of oral carcinoma. Ig Sanita Pubbl. 2018;74(3):249–63.
20. Sanger JR, Matloub HS, Yousif NJ. Sequential connection of flaps: a logical approach to customized mandibular reconstruction. Am J Surg. 1990;160:402–4.
21. Soutar DS, Widdowson WP. Immediate reconstruction of the mandible using a vascularized segment of radius. Head Neck Surg. 1986;8(4):232–46.
22. Yoo J, Dowthwaite SA, Fung K, Franklin J, Nichols A. A new angle to mandibular reconstruction: the scapular tip free flap. Head Neck. 2013;35(7):980–6.

Maxilla: Types I–IV

Giorgio De Santis, Pier Francesco Nocini,
and Luigi Chiarini

Maxillary defects resulting from tumour or trauma can lead to severe cosmetic and functional deformities. Maxillary bone provides height and width to the midface, contributing greatly to aesthetic facial contour, and moreover separates the oral from the nasal and orbital cavities; it also provides skeletal support to the orbital contents. Owing to these anatomical factors, maxillary defects affect speech, swallowing and mastication and can cause dystopia.

As a consequence, maxillary reconstruction is extraordinarily challenging and is still an evolving art when compared to the reconstruction of the mandible.

Maxillectomy defects become very difficult when critical structures such as the orbit, the globe and the cranial base are resected, and often the use of distant tissues becomes essential in this case.

The loss of the vertical component causes more of an aesthetic problem, while the horizontal component loss results in greater functional deficits.

The primary goal of maxillary reconstruction is functional preservation, supporting of the orbital contents, and optimization of feeding and speech. A secondary goal is aesthetic restoration of patient's appearance with adequate midfacial projection and vertical facial height.

It is not necessary to reconstruct all the walls of the maxilla, but it is necessary to restore midface contour, to provide orbital floor support and to replace the missing alveolar bone as to a base for dental implants.

G. De Santis (✉)
Plastic and Reconstructive Surgery Unit, University Hospital of Modena, Modena, Italy
e-mail: desantis.giorgio@unimore.it

P. F. Nocini
Division of Oral and Maxillo-Facial Surgery, University Hospital of Verona, Verona, Italy
e-mail: pierfrancesco.nocini@univr.it

L. Chiarini
Cranio-Maxillo-Facial Surgery Unit, University Hospital of Modena, Modena, Italy
e-mail: luigi.chiarini@unimore.it

Various classification systems have tried to look at the defects from their functional and/or aesthetic effects. We briefly describe the maxillary reconstructive principles related to specific defects, referring to the classification proposed by P. G. Cordeiro. This classification is based on the number of walls resected, the need for the palatal closure and the need for orbital reconstruction (see chapter "Classification System for Maxillectomy Defects") [1].

The maxilla can be described as a six-sided box or hexahedrium [2, 3].

The roof of the maxilla is the floor of the orbit and supports the ocular globe. The body of the maxilla consists of the anterior, posterior, medial and lateral walls and provides midfacial projection and vertical facial height. The floor of the maxilla corresponds to the hard palate and is essential for mastication, speech and deglutition.

Many approaches have been explored for the reconstruction of the maxilla. Among the various techniques, free fibula flaps are widely used and have achieved satisfactory long-term results.

The osteocutaneous fibula flap can provide, in particular, a favourable foundation for three-dimensional reconstruction of maxillary defects because recreating the infraorbital rim and the orbital floor is essential to successfully maintain the position of the ocular globe [4–8].

It is also useful in the maxillary arch to provide anterior projection of the midface and bone stock for osseointegrated implants [7, 9].

In our opinion, the osteocutaneous fibula flap is particularly suitable in maxilla defects in which the basal bone and alveolar process are absent (lack of the bone floor of the maxillary sinus and the nasal cavity) and an implant-borne prosthetic rehabilitation is planned. Multiple osteotomies for contouring the fibula shaft are needed considering the three-dimensional complexity of the upper jaw; we recommend piezosurgical device for remodelling procedure. Anesi et al. (2018) demonstrated that osteotomies performed using piezosurgical devices show more advanced stages of bone healing compared with rotary instruments. Moreover, even more powerful devices (output power of 75 W) do not alter the process of bone healing [10–12].

G. De Santis et al. (eds.), *Atlas of Mandibular and Maxillary Reconstruction with the Fibula Flap*,
https://doi.org/10.1007/978-3-030-10684-3_6

Type I Defects

Type I defects (limited or partial maxillectomy) include resection of one or two walls of the maxilla, excluding the palate. The anterior and medial walls are the most commonly resected. The resection will often include the soft tissue and skin of the cheek and even the lips, nose and eyelids.

According to Cordeiro, the radial forearm free flap can provide good external skin coverage and minimal bulk while allowing multiple skin islands. If the orbital rim or orbital floor has been resected, non-vascularized bone grafts can provide the needed support. When subcutaneous tissue is thin, an anterolateral thigh flap might be an appropriate choice as well.

Type II Defects

Type II defects (subtotal maxillectomy) include resection of the lower five walls of maxilla, including the palate, but sparing the orbital floor (roof of maxilla), and these defects may be further subdivided into type IIA defects, which include the loss of less than 50% of the transverse palate, and type IIB defects, which include greater than 50% of the transverse palate and/or the anterior arch of the maxilla.

Type IIA Defects

Reconstruction of type IIA defects could involve an oral obturator or a skin graft or free flap. For Cordeiro et al., the flap of choice is the radial forearm fasciocutaneous free flap [7].

If the alveolar process has to be restored for implant-borne prosthetic rehabilitation, in our opinion, the osteocutaneous fibula flap is suitable for a type IIA defect reconstruction (Figs. 1–6). The soft tissue management is complicated, as the skin island flap has to be smaller than the defect in order to avoid prolapse into the oral cavity. Remodelling and thinning of the island's skin is also described as the healing is complete.

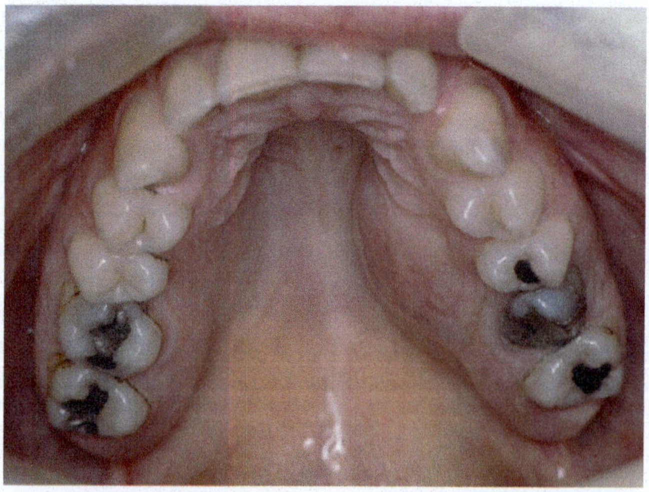

Fig. 1 Left palatal swelling due to an adenoid cystic carcinoma developed by palatal minor salivary glands

Type IIB Defects

Reconstruction of this defect required an osteocutaneous free flap, as an obturator could not provide an adequate support to the upper lip. Moreover, the bone segment (fibula flap in particular) may be used for implant-anchored prosthetic rehabilitation (Figs. 7–11). Radial osteocutaneous sandwich flap is also described [6].

Type III Defects

Type III defects (total maxillectomy) include resection of all six walls of the maxilla with orbital content preservation (type IIIA) or with orbital exenteration (type IIIB).

Type IIIA Defects

After the resection of all six walls of the maxilla as a consequence of advanced cancer, we had medium–large volume and medium–large surface area defects [13].

The purpose was to support the globe (in order to avoid dystopia, which could result in enophthalmos, hypophthalmos and diplopia), obliterate communication between the orbit and nasopharynx and obtain dental rehabilitation. The reconstructive task of providing adequate support of the orbit is therefore technically more demanding than when even the orbital content is resected.

An osteomyocutaneous fibula flap offered a good orbital rim and floor reconstruction, preserved the malar eminence and maintained the projection of the upper midface (Figs. 12–14) [14].

Type IIIB Defects

Type IIIB defects involve resection of all six walls of the maxilla, including exenteration of the orbital contents (Figs. 14–20).

Soft tissue pedicled flaps, such as the temporalis flap, passed into the orbit through osteotomized lateral orbital wall are useful in patients who cannot undergo free-tissue transfer [15].

Latissimus dorsi flap, rectus abdominis free flap and deep inferior epigastric perforator flap have the volume required to refill the midface contour and to seal the nasal fossa and oral cavity [16].

If orbitozygomatic contour is resected, a vascularized bony flap can restore midface projection with or without a further soft tissue transfer. Free fibula flap, iliac crest free flap and scapula free flap are well described in the literature [17].

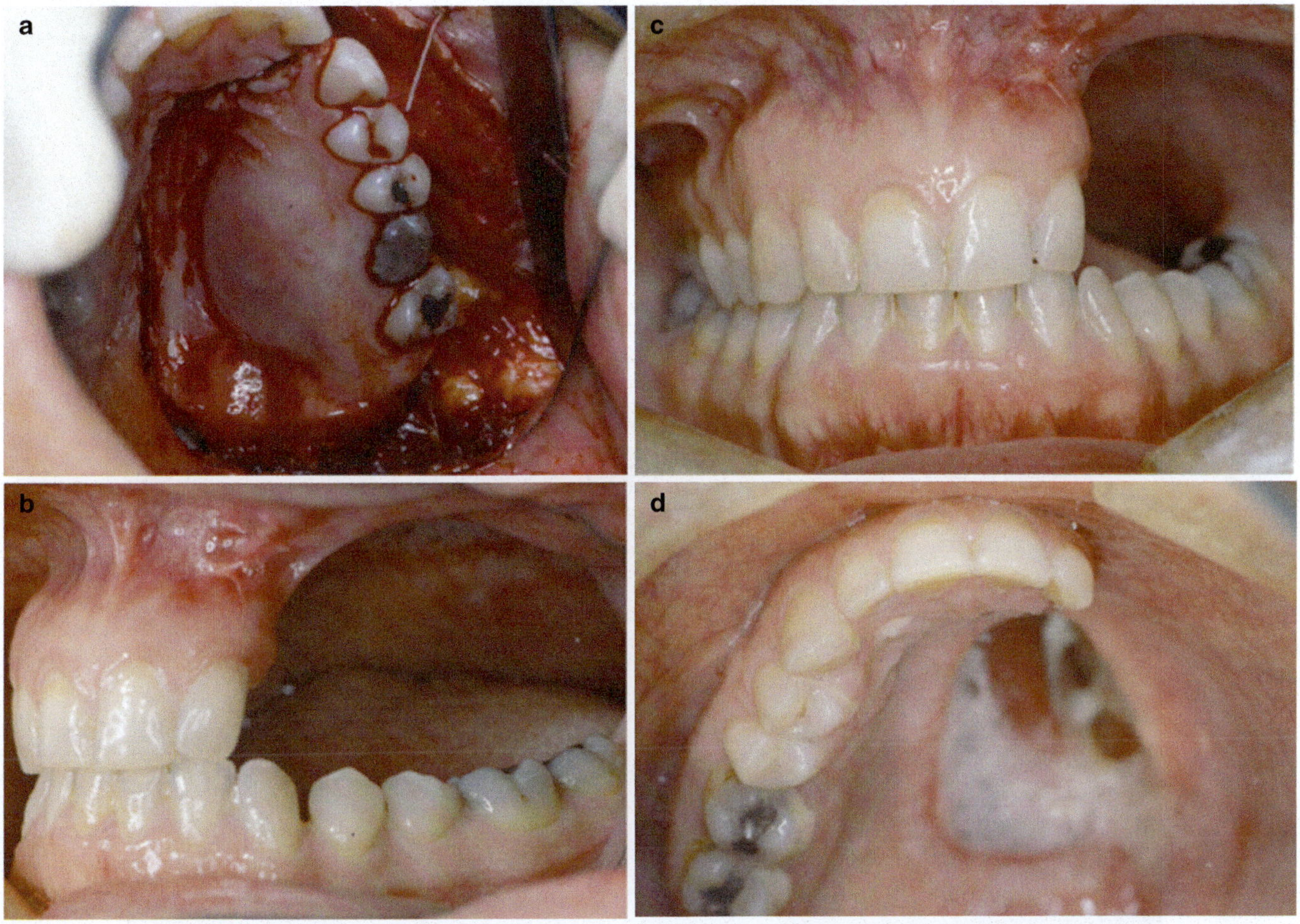

Fig. 2 (**a**) A low posterior maxillectomy was performed, causing a type IIA defect (according to P. G. Cordeiro's classification). (**b–d**) Delayed lateral, frontal and palatal view of the intraoral defect. Histological findings confirmed clear (negative) resection margins. Therefore, delayed maxillary reconstruction was planned

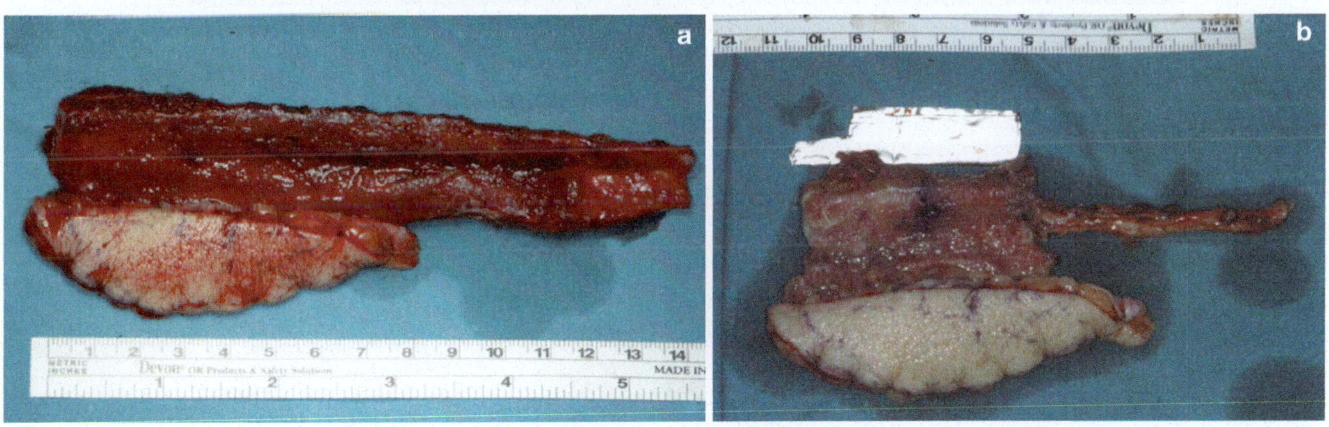

Fig. 3 (**a**) Osteo-septo-cutaneous fibula flap was harvested. (**b**) Drawing with a marking for fibula flap shaping according to defect dimension

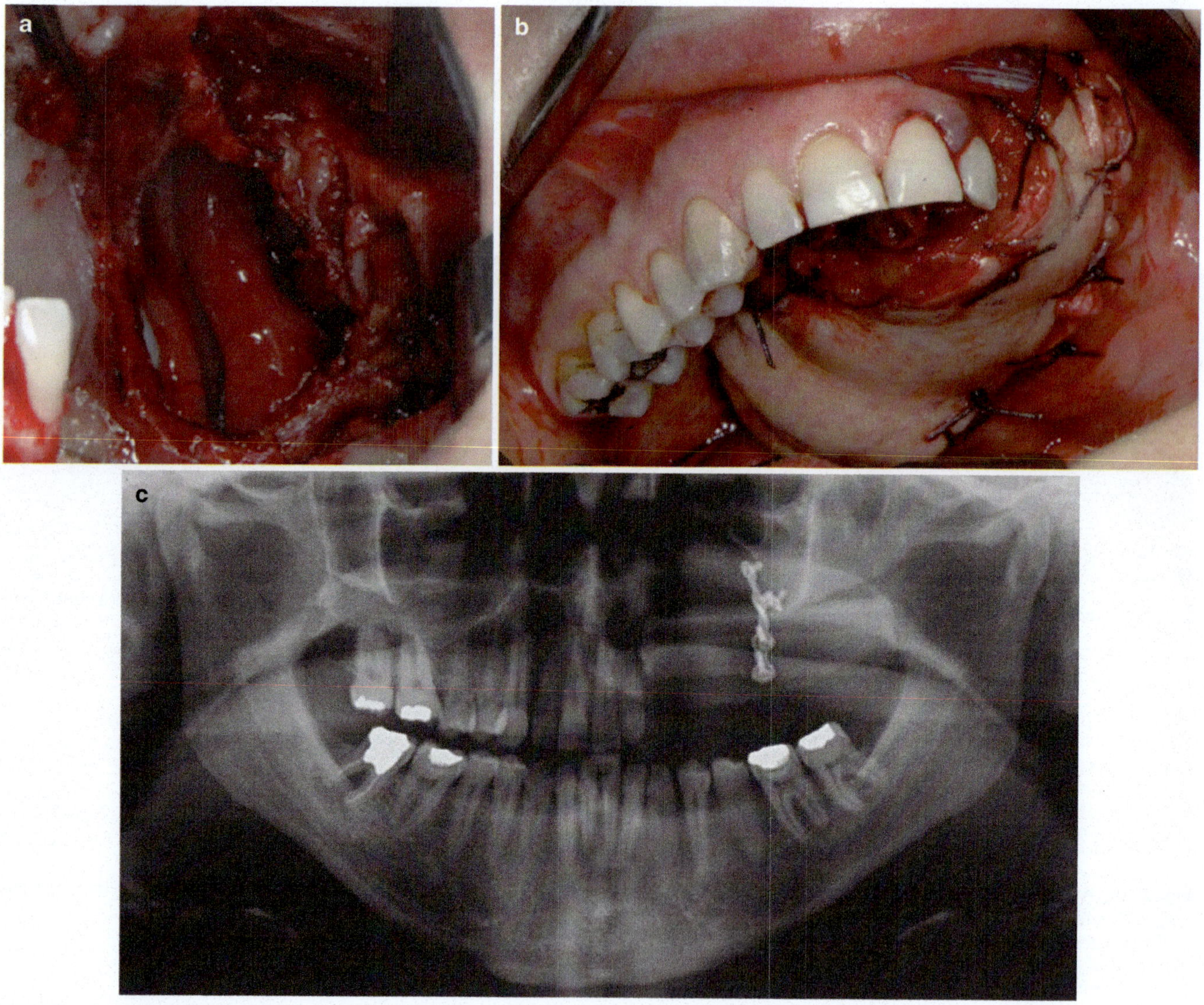

Fig. 4 (**a**) The surgical margins of the defect are ready for flap insetting. (**b**) The Fibula flap was fixed and the skin island sutured to the natural mucosa lining. (**c**) Postoperative orthopantomograph

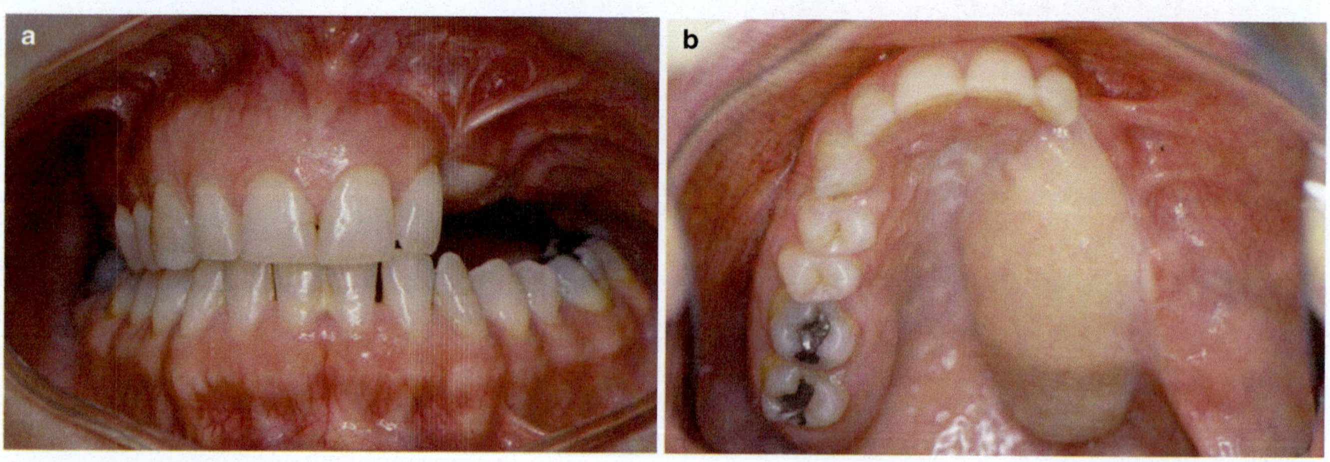

Fig. 5 (**a** and **b**) Postoperative intraoral view

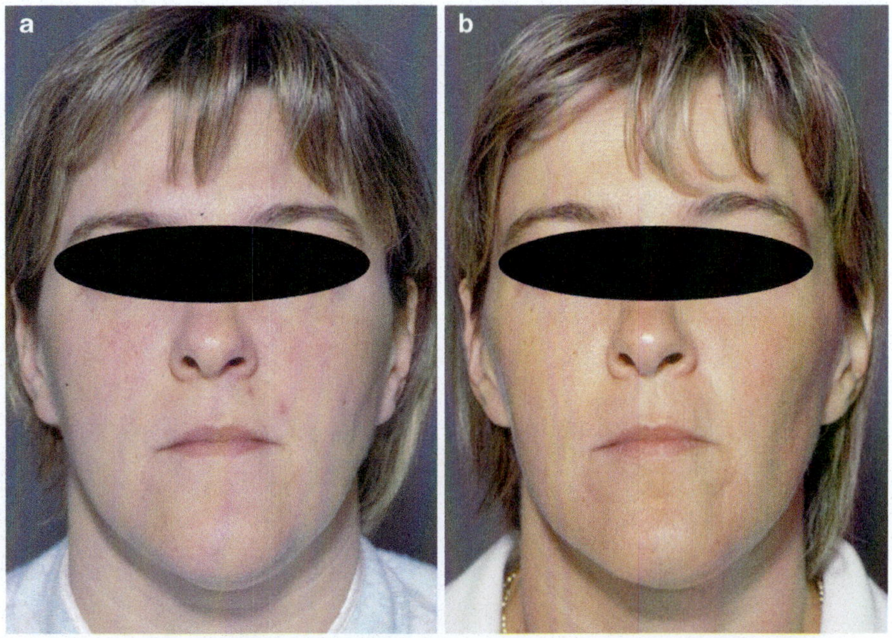

Fig. 6 (**a** and **b**) Preoperative and postoperative frontal view of the patient in Figs. 1–5

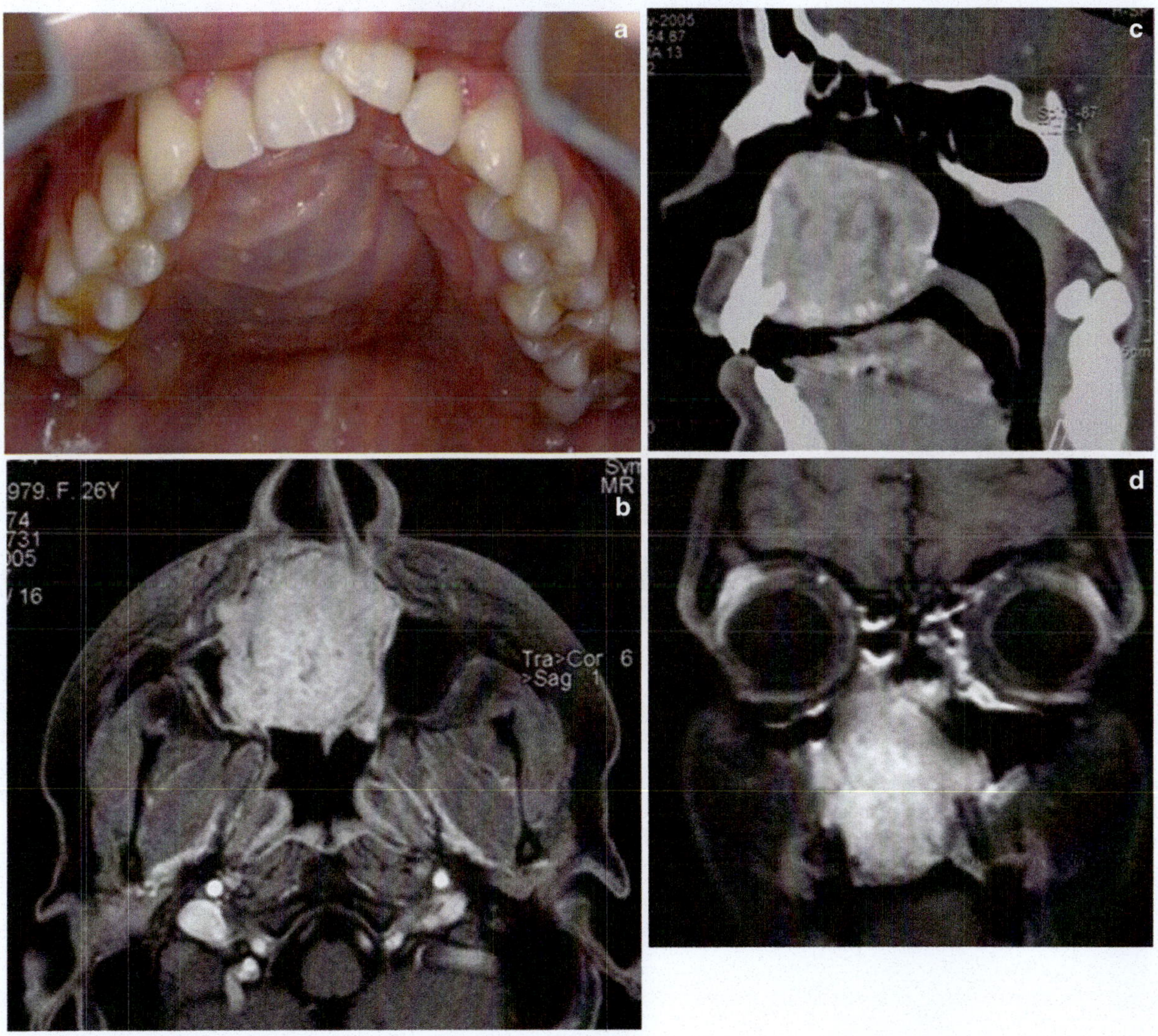

Fig. 7 (**a**) Malignant myoepithelioma of the palate in a 27-year-old girl. (**b**) Preoperative MRI: the malignancy filled the nasal fossa. (**c**) Bone erosion of the palate. (**d**) Both orbital floors are not interested by the neoplasia

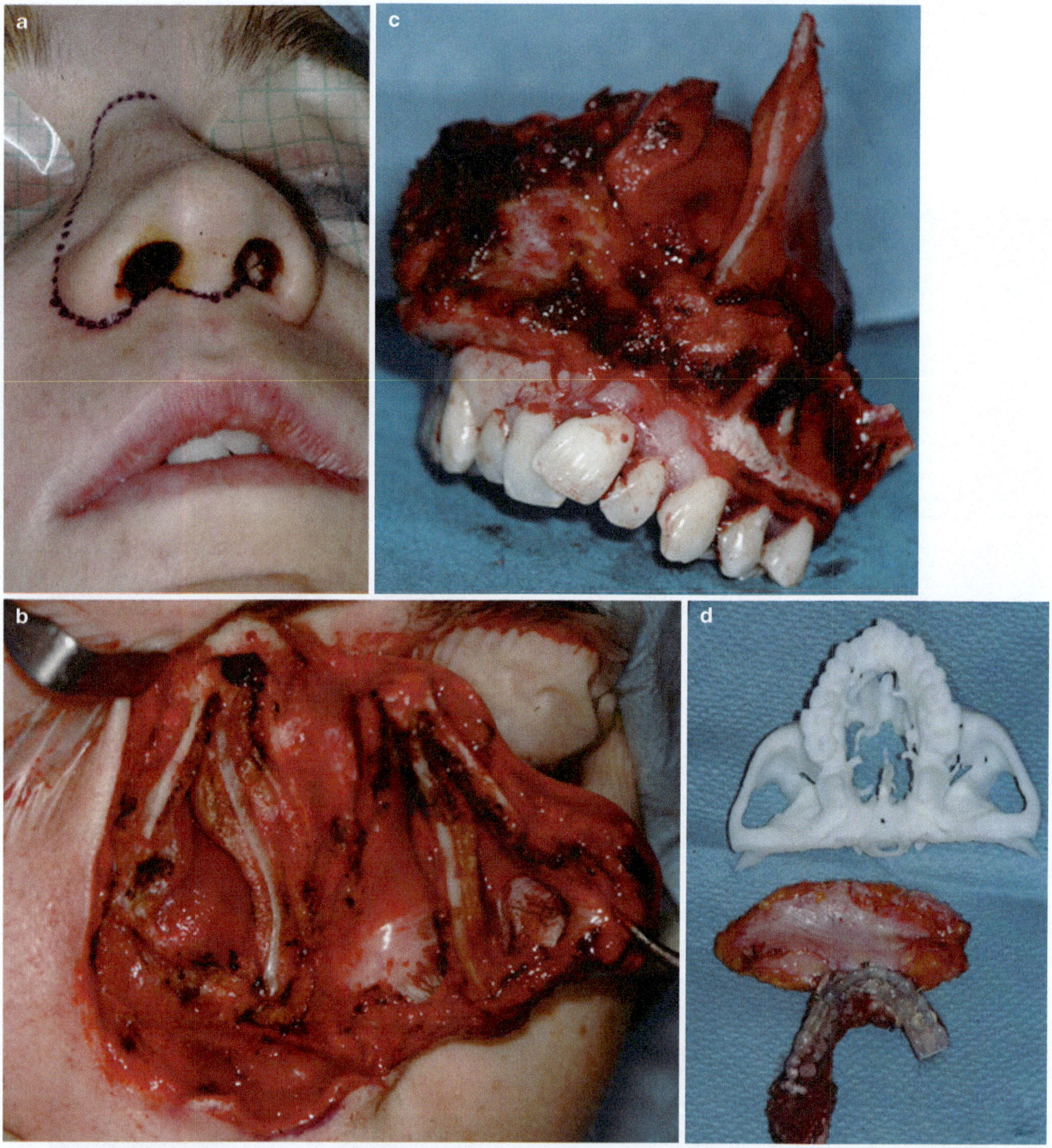

Fig. 8 (**a** and **b**) Lateral rhinotomy and intraoral degloving were chosen for approach to the tumour. (**c**) Bilateral maxillectomy with orbital wall preservation can be classified as a type IIB defects (according to P. G. Cordeiro's classification). (**d**) A stereolithographic model was used to shape the osteo-septo-cutaneous fibula flap

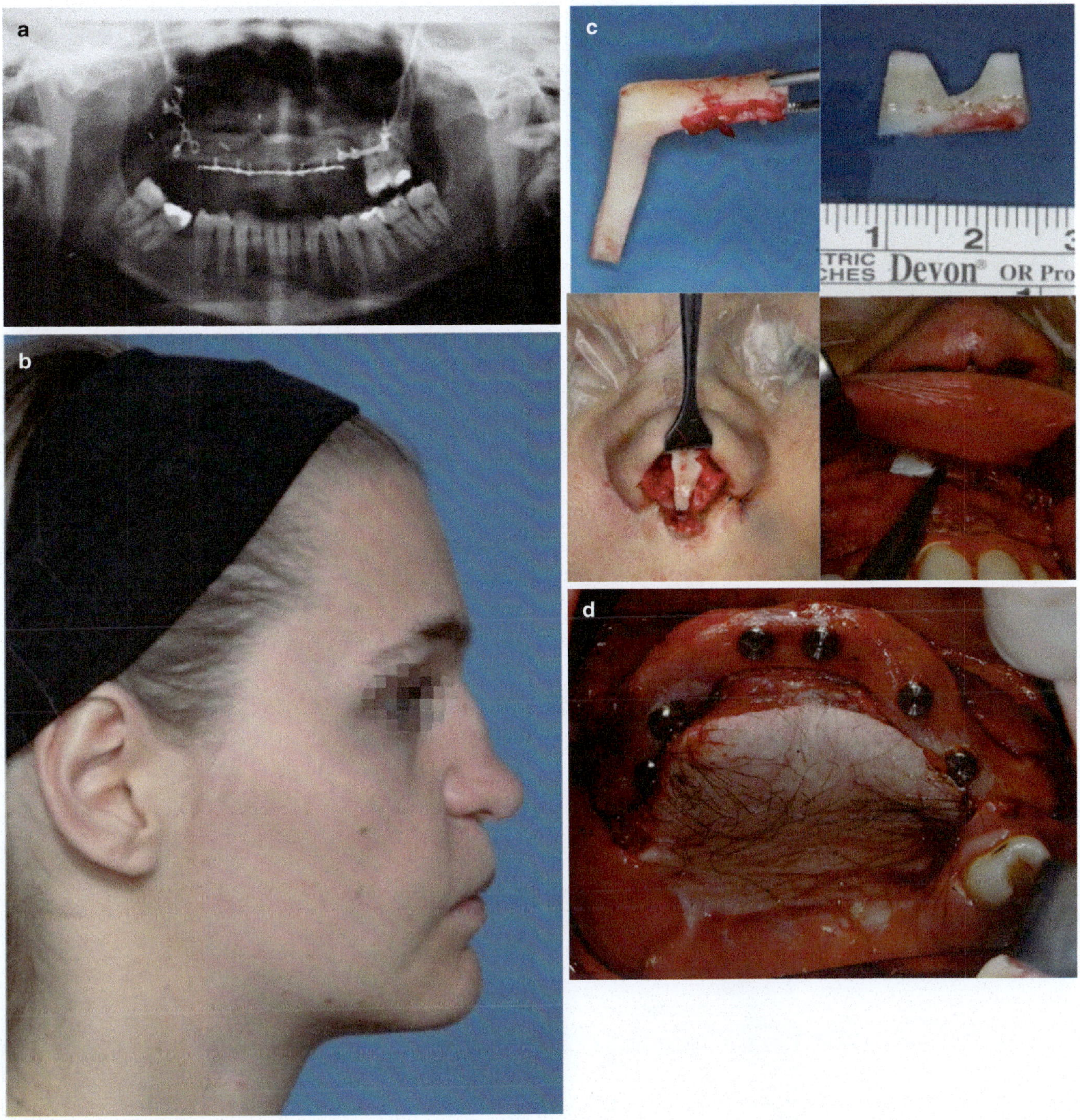

Fig. 9 (**a**) Postoperative orthopantomograph showing adequate restoration of upper alveolar arch. (**b–d**) Because of nasal deformity due to nasal septum resection, nose reconstruction by costal rib graft was carried out 6 months later. Contemporary titanium plate removal and endosseous dental implant positioning

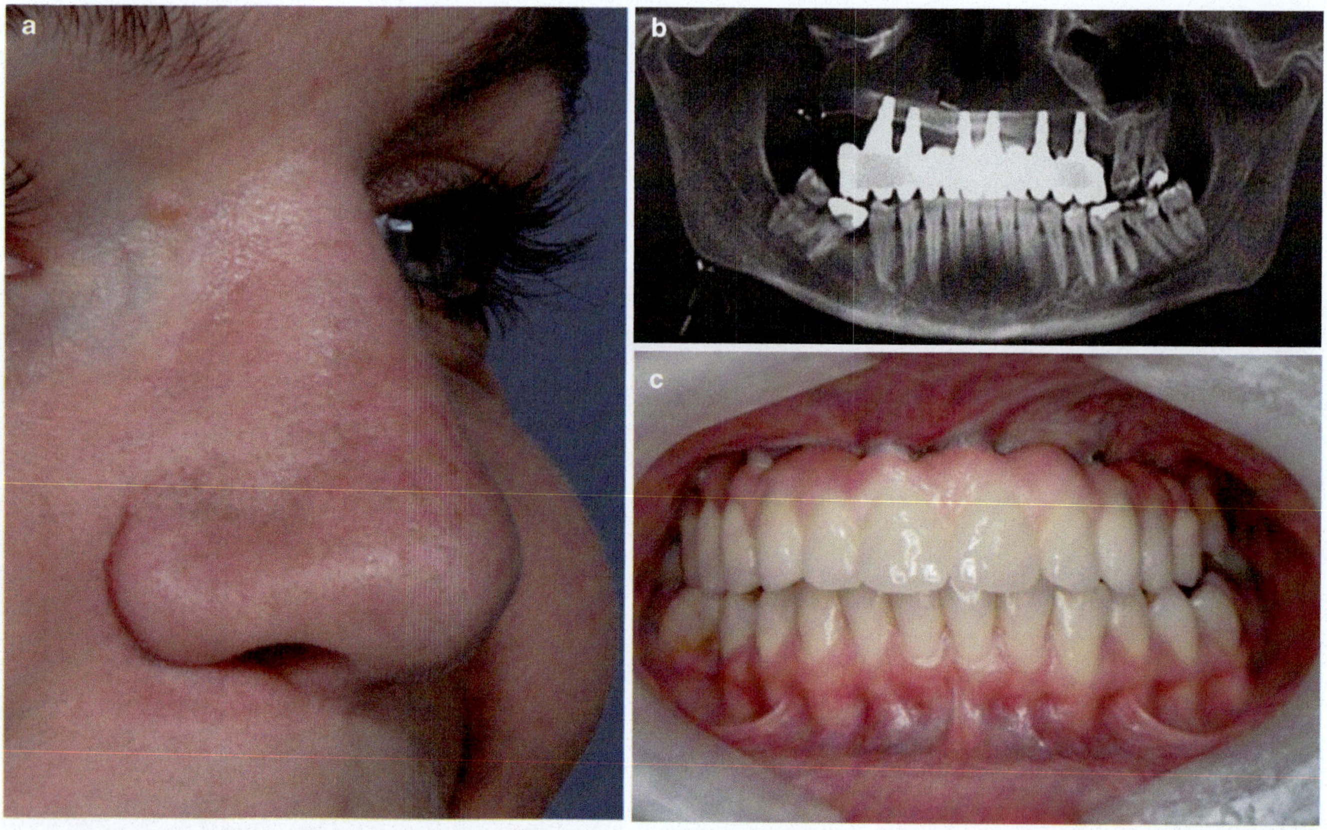

Fig. 10 (**a**) Nasal pyramid projection was restored. (**b**) Postoperative orthopantomograph with implant-borne dental prosthesis. (**c**) Complete dental rehabilitation

Fig. 11 (**a** and **b**) Preoperative and postoperative frontal view of the patient in Figs. 7–10

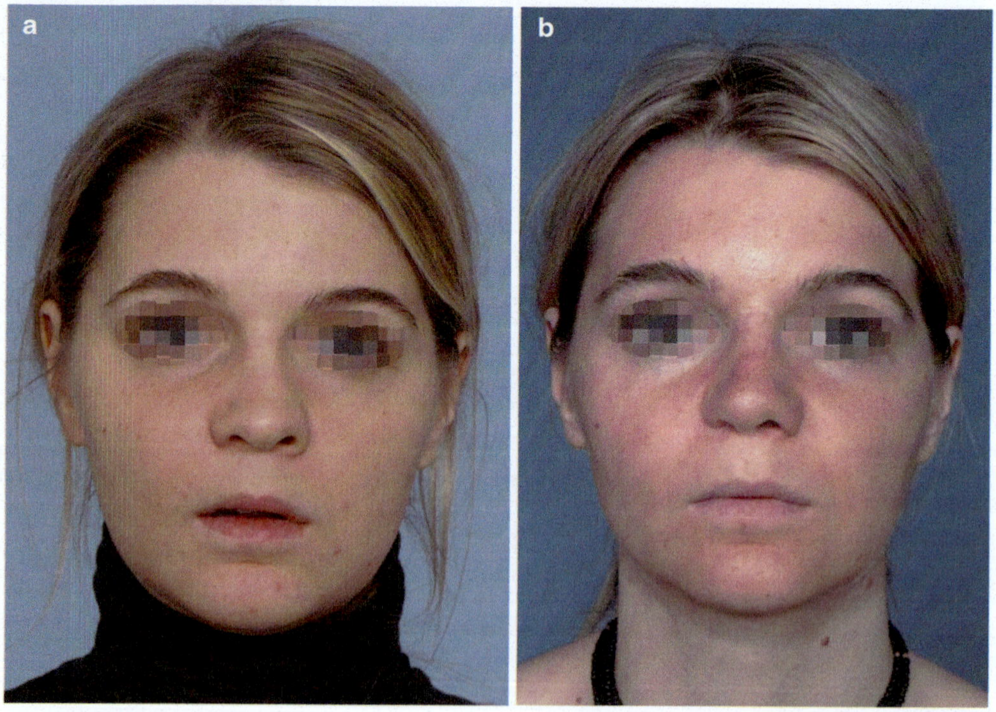

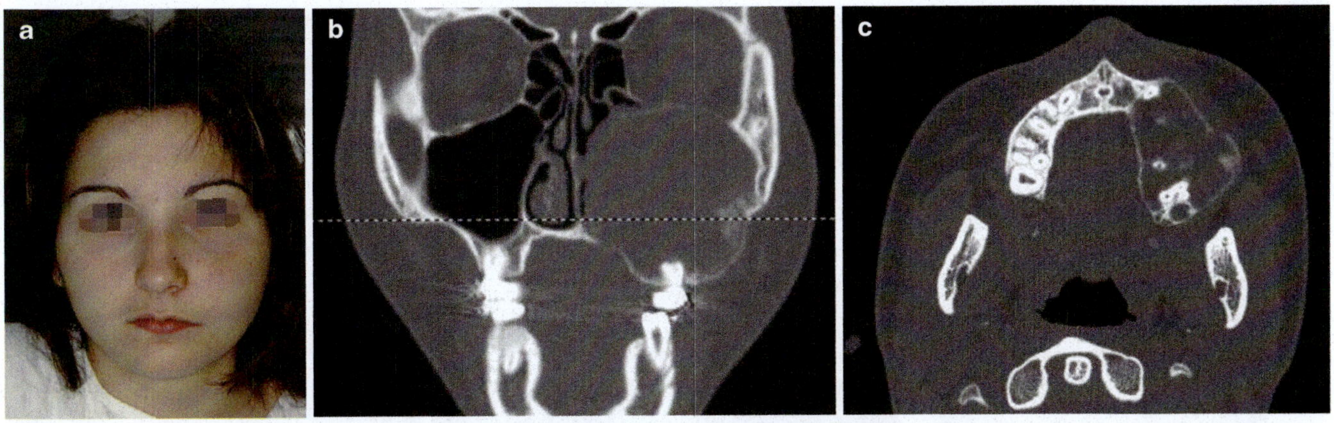

Fig. 12 (**a**) 12-year-old patient, preoperative frontal view. Note dystopia of left eye and bulking maxillary mass. (**b** and **c**) Axial and coronal images of a psammomatous ossifying fibroma involving whole left maxillary bone and even orbital floor

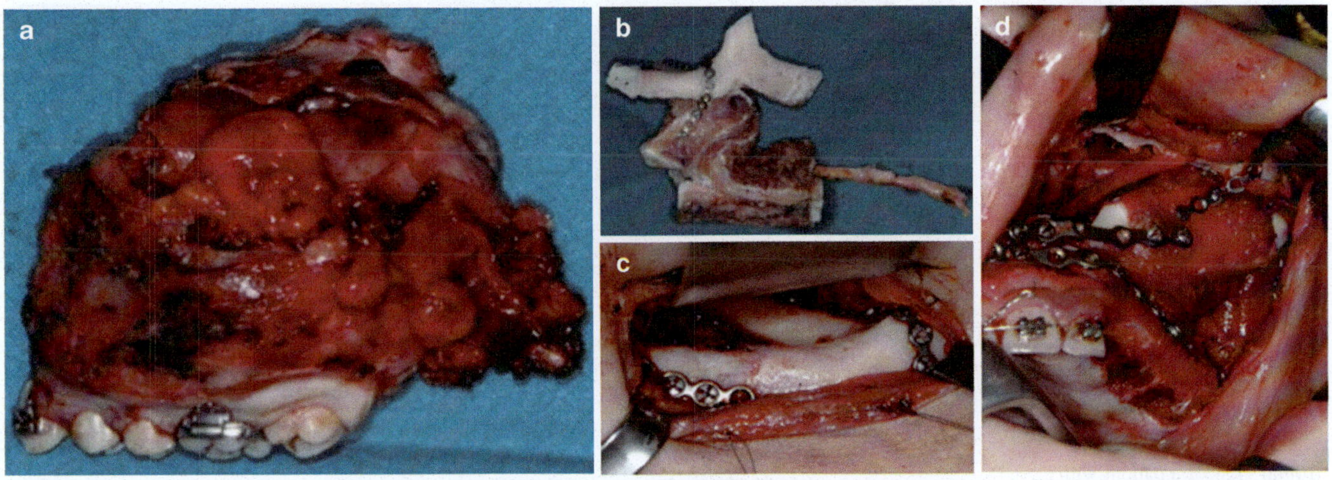

Fig. 13 Intraoperative images. (**a**) Surgical specimen after total left maxillectomy including the floor of the orbit which gave to a type IIIA defect (according to P. G. Cordeiro's classification). (**b**) Fibula flap shaping in three bony segments, synthesized with the previously osteotomized inferior orbital rim and zygomatic bone. (**c**) Fibula flap insetting with orbital floor reconstruction. (**d**) The fibula muscle is sutured to the palatal mucosa with resorbable suture to create a watertight seal

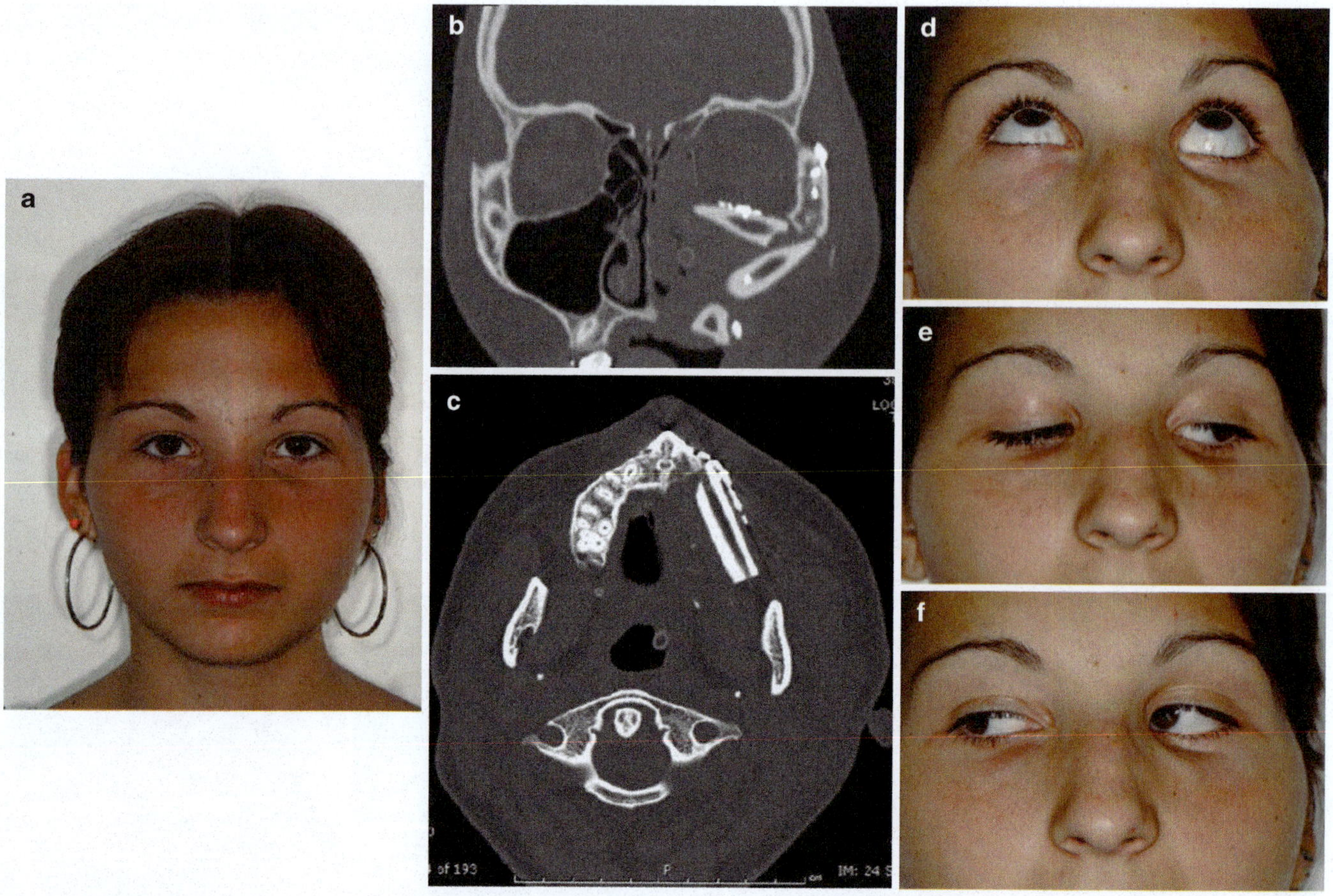

Fig. 14 (**a**) Postoperative frontal view of the patient. (**b** and **c**) Radiological post-treatment images showing the fibula segments well aligned and held stable by plates. (**d–f**) No extraocular muscle deficit were present as healing was completed

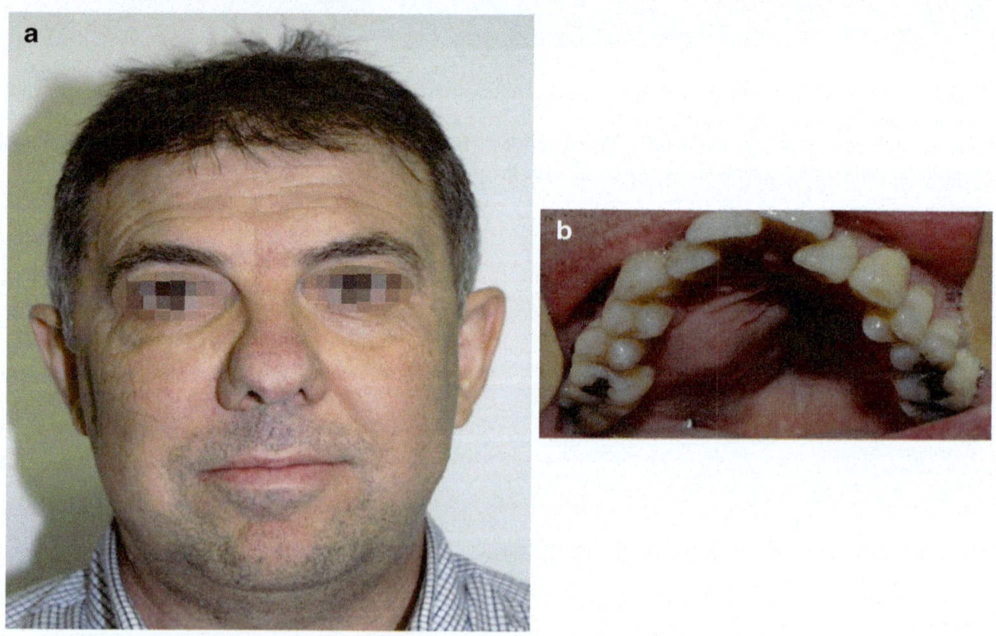

Fig. 15 (**a**) Preoperative frontal view of a patient with an adenoid cystic carcinoma; (**b**) note right intraoral palatal bulking

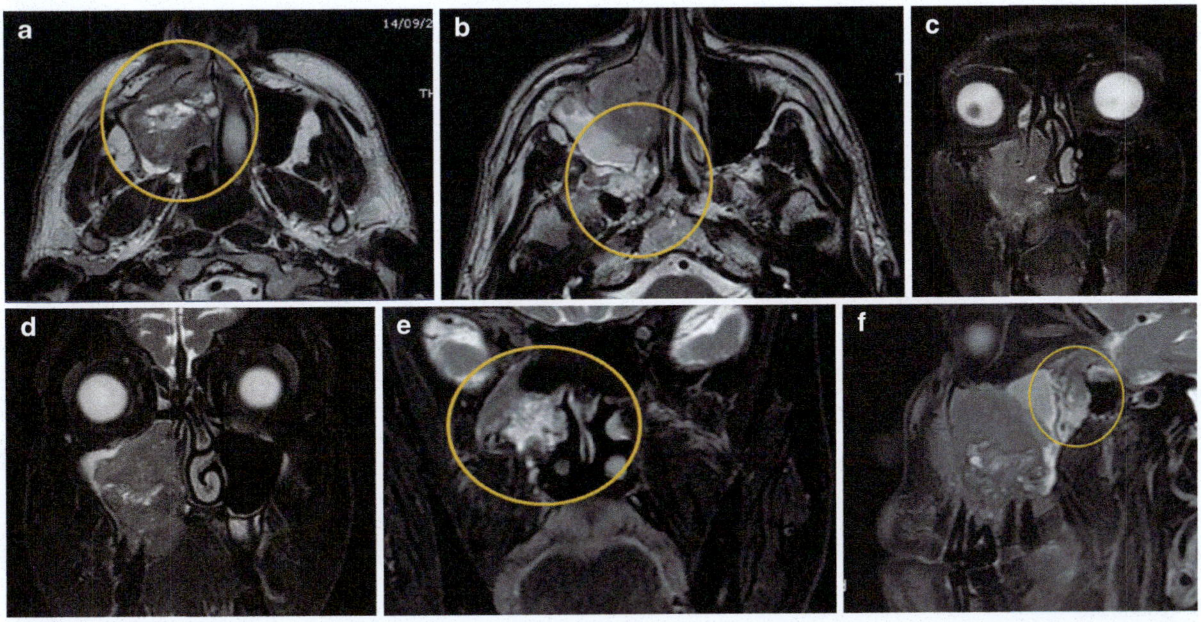

Fig. 16 (**a–f**) Preoperative MRI images showing wide spread of the malignancy into the maxillary sinus, the nasal fossa, the pterygopalatine fossa and the right orbit

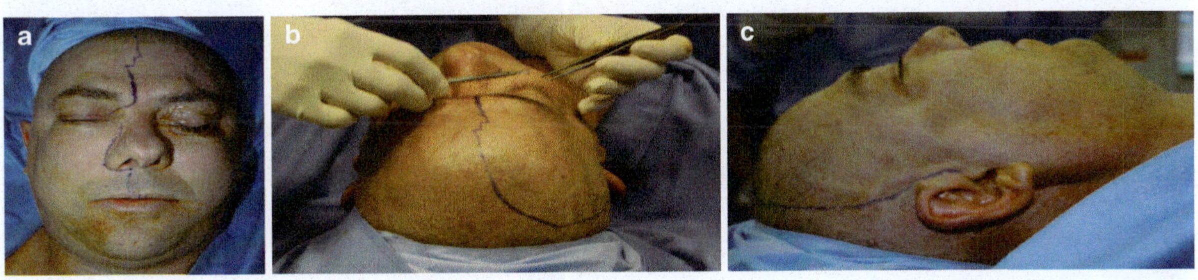

Fig. 17 (**a–c**) Transfacial approach was chosen: Weber-Fergusson incision with subciliary and supraciliary extension, continued upwards in a unilateral hemicoronal approach

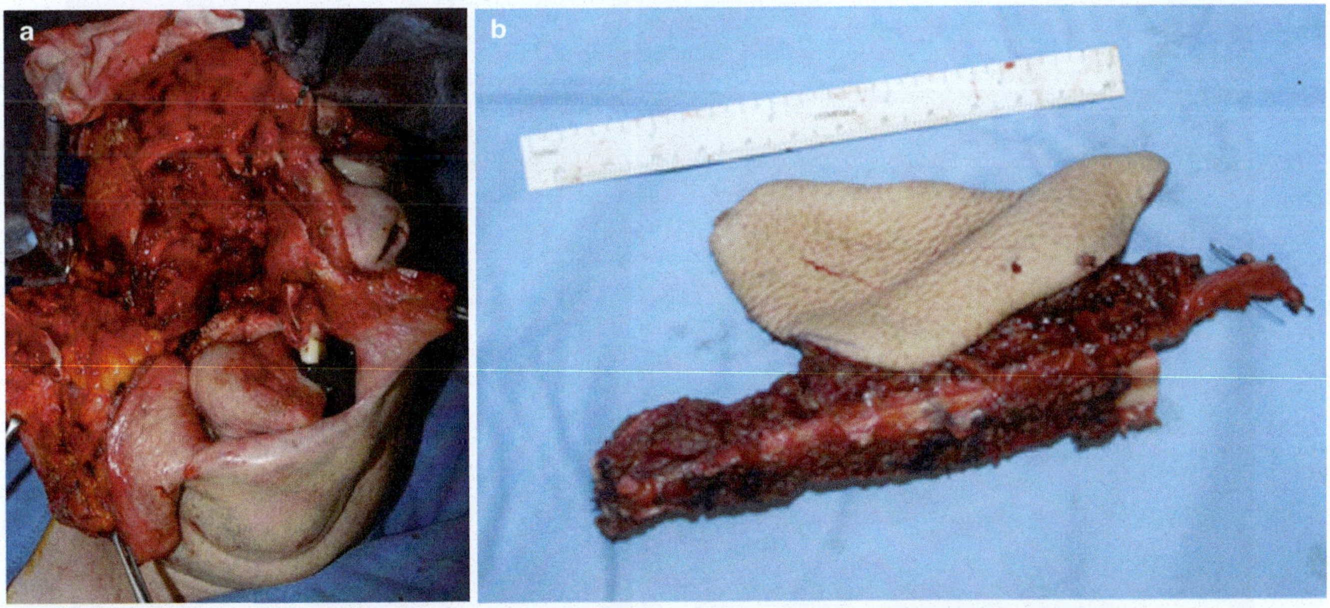

Fig. 18 (**a**) Osteomyocutaneous fibula flap harvested. (**b**) Wide defect following extirpation of right maxillary adenoid cystic carcinoma involving the orbital floor and content, maxilla, palate, alveolar arch and pterygoid plates. Orbitomaxillectomy defect was classifiable as type IV defects (according to P. G. Cordeiro's classification) (**c**) Osteomyocutaneous fibula flap shaped. (**d**) Insetting of fibula flap and right temporalis muscle flap used to fill in the defect after orbital exenteration

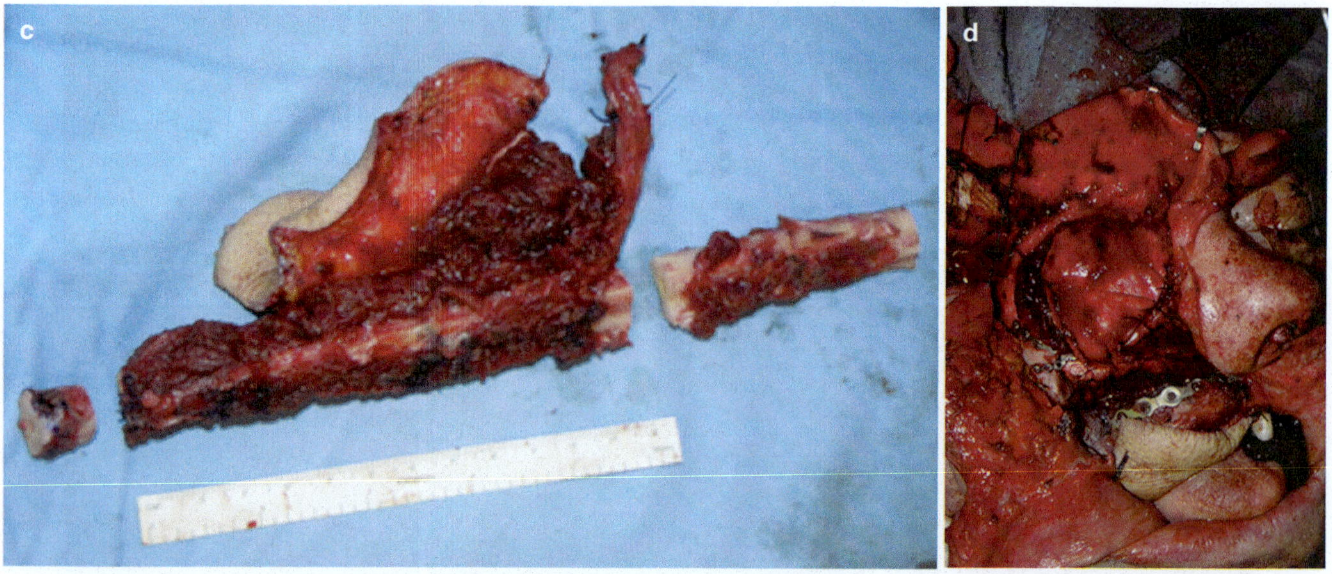

Fig. 18 (contimed)

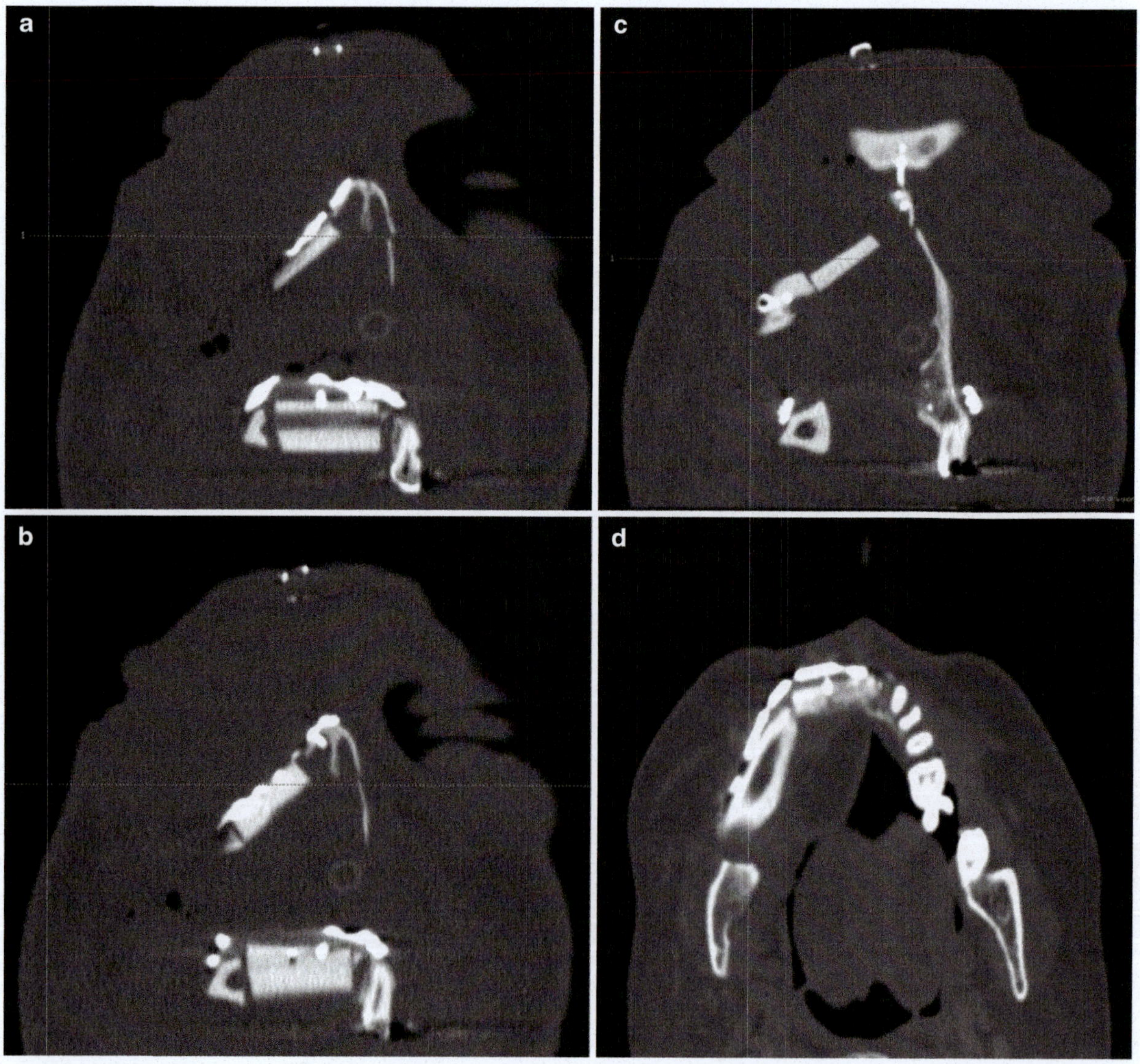

Fig. 19 (**a–d**) Postoperative CT scans. Fibula flap restores both the alveolar arch and the orbital rim and floor

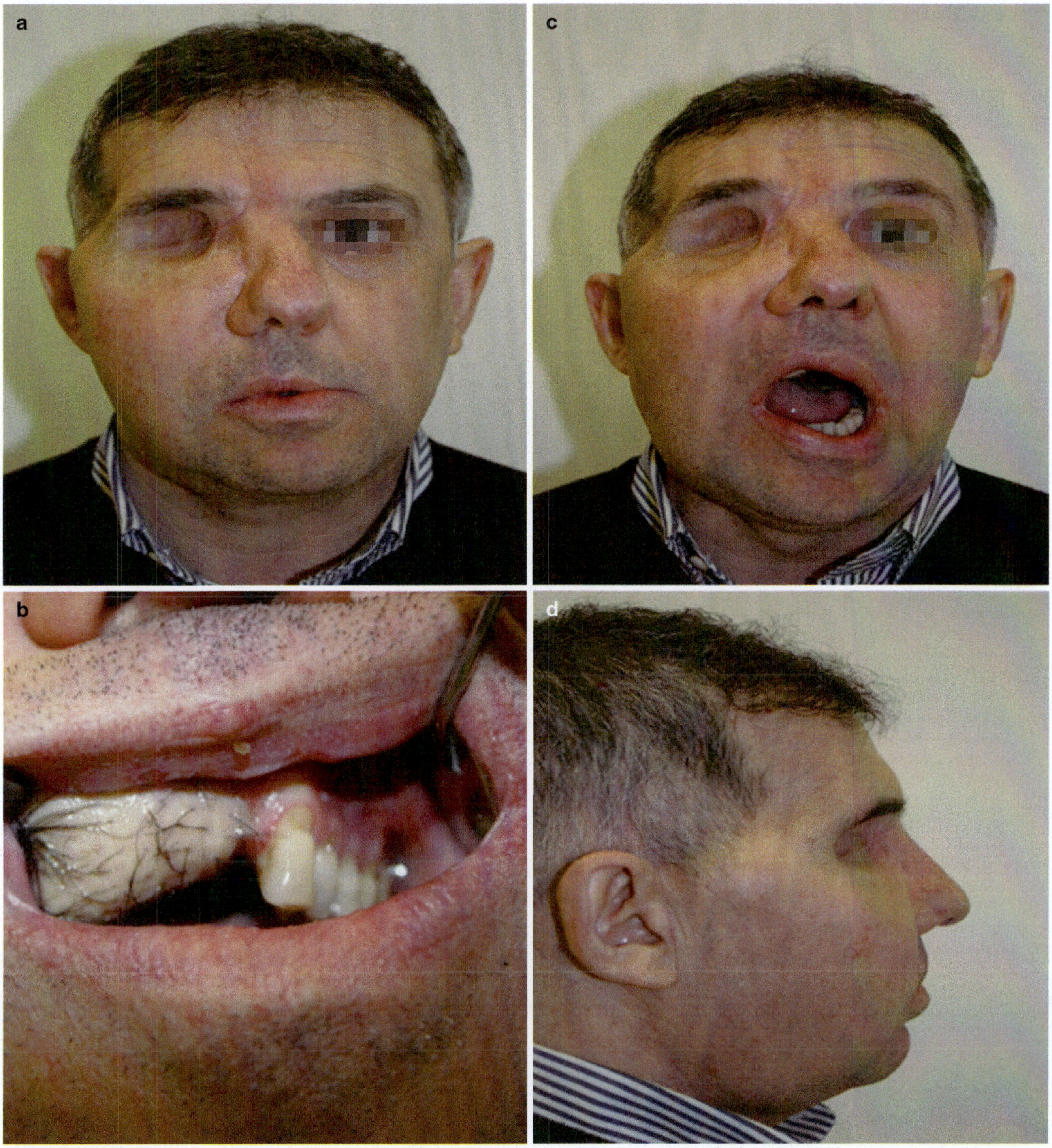

Fig. 20 (**a**) One-year post-treatment frontal view of the patient after surgery. Adjuvant hadron therapy was performed. (**b**) Intraoral view of the fibula flap skin island used for intraoral reconstruction. Note hair growth on the skin paddle. (**c** and **d**) Pictures showing patient's midface projection preservation following large resection. Implant-borne prosthetic rehabilitation was not carried out, because a relapse occurred

Type IV Defects

Finally, type IV defects (orbitomaxillectomy) include resection of the orbital contents and the upper five walls of the maxilla, with preservation of the palate. The flap of choice is the rectus abdominis flap or latissimus dorsi flap.

For sealing of nasal fossa and paranasal sinuses, a bulky myocutaneous flap is needed, i.e. latissimus dorsi flap, rectus abdominis free flap and deep inferior epigastric perforator flap [18].

For radical orbital exenteration cavities with resection of overlying skin and bony malar eminence, osteocutaneous scapula flap was used [19].

Fibula osteomyocutaneous flap or deep circumflex iliac artery-based iliac crest flap can be used together with a myocutaneous flap (i.e. latissimus dorsi flap, anterolateral thigh flap, rectus abdominis free flap and deep inferior epigastric perforator flap) [20].

References

1. Cordeiro PG, Chen CM. A 15-year review of midface reconstruction after total and subtotal maxillectomy: part I. algorithm and outcomes. Plast Reconstr Surg. 2012;129(1):124–36.
2. Wells MD, Luce EA. Reconstruction of midfacial defects after surgical resection of malignancies. Clin Plast Surg. 1995;22(1):79–89.
3. Swartz WM, Banis JC, Newton ED, Ramasastry SS, Jones NF, Acland R. The osteocutaneous scapular flap for mandibular and maxillary reconstruction. Plast Reconstr Surg. 1986;77(4):530–45.
4. Sadove RC, Powell LA. Simultaneous maxillary and mandibular reconstruction with one free osteocutaneous flap. Plast Reconstr Surg. 1993;92(1):141–6.
5. Swartz WM, Banis JC. Orbital maxillary reconstruction. In: Swartz WM, Banis JC, editors. Head and neck microsurgery. Baltimore: Williams & Wilkins; 1990. p. 225.
6. Cordeiro PG, Bacilious N, Schantz S, Spiro R. The radial forearm osteocutaneous "sandwich" free flap for reconstruction of the bilateral subtotal maxillectomy defect. Ann Plast Surg. 1998;40(4):397–402.
7. Cordeiro PG, Santamaria E, Kraus DH, Strong EW, Shah JP. Reconstruction of total maxillectomy defects with preservation of the orbital contents. Plast Reconstr Surg. 1998;102(6):1874–84. discussion 1885–7.
8. Anesi A, Pollastri G, Barberini S, Ferrari C, Sarconi G, Chiarini L. Retrospective analysis of orbital floor fractures: our clinical experience. Italian J Oral Maxillofac Surg. 2013;24(2):63–8.
9. Kyutoku S, Tsuji H, Inoue T, Kawakami K, Han F, Ogawa Y. Experience with the rectus abdominis myocutaneous flap with vascularized hard tissue for immediate orbitofacial reconstruction. Plast Reconstr Surg. 1999;103(2):395–402.
10. Anesi A, Ferretti M, Cavani F, Salvatori R, Bianchi M, Russo A, Chiarini L, Palumbo C. Structural and ultrastructural analyses of bone regeneration in rabbit cranial osteotomy: Piezosurgery versus traditional osteotomes. J Craniomaxillofac Surg. 2018;46(1):107–18. https://doi.org/10.1016/j.jcms.2017.10.004. Epub 2017 Oct 12.
11. Turra M, Bertossi D, Bissolotti G, Anesi A, Chiarini L, Nocini PF. O.095 Genioplasty with piezosurgery. J Craniomaxillofac Surg. 2008;36(Suppl1):S24. https://doi.org/10.1016/S1010-5182(08)71219-8.
12. Chiarini L, Albanese M, Anesi A, Galzignato PF, Mortellaro C, Nocini P, Bertossi D. Surgical treatment of unilateral condylar hyperplasia with piezosurgery. J Craniofac Surg. 2014;25(3):808–10. https://doi.org/10.1097/SCS.0000000000000699.
13. Marella GL, Raschellà F, Solinas M, Mutolo P, Potenza S, Milano F, Mauriello S, Caggiano B, Rondinelli P, Anesi A, Migaldi M. The diagnostic delay of oral carcinoma. Ig Sanita Pubbl. 2018;74(3):249–63.
14. Lundgren TK, Pignatti M, Halle M, Boscaini G, Skogh AC, Chiarini L, De Santis G. Composite orbital reconstruction using the vascularized segmentalized osteo-fascio-cutaneous fibula flap. J Plast Reconstr Aesthet Surg. 2016;69(2):255–61. https://doi.org/10.1016/j.bjps.2015.10.012. Epub 2015 Oct 26.
15. Muzaffar AR, Adams WP, Hartog JM, et al. Maxillary reconstruction: functional and aesthetic considerations. Plast Reconstr Surg. 1999;104:2172–83.
16. Shestak KC, Schusterman MA, Jones NF, Johnson JT. Immediate microvascular reconstruction of combined palatal and midfacial defects using soft tissue only. Microsurgery. 1988;9(2):128–31.
17. Futran ND, Mendez E. Developments in reconstruction of midface and maxilla. Lancet Oncol. 2006;7(3):249–58. Review.
18. Cordeiro PG, Santamaria E. A classification system and algorithm for reconstruction of maxillectomy and midfacial defects plastic and reconstructive surgery. Plast Reconstr Surg. 2000;105:2331–46.
19. Chepeha DB, Moyer JS, Bradford CR, et al. Osseocutaneous radial forearm free tissue transfer for repair of complex midfacial defects. Arch Otolaryngol Head Neck Surg. 2005;131:513–7.
20. Brown JS, Jones DC, Summerwill A, Rogers SN, Howell RA, Cawood JI, et al. Vascularized iliac crest with internal oblique muscle for immediate reconstruction after maxillectomy. Br J Oral Maxillofac Surg. 2002;40:183–90.

Bone Augmentation

Pier Francesco Nocini, Alexandre Anesi, and Andrea Fior

The main limitation of the free fibula flap reconstruction is bone height that is insufficient for restoring both the skeletal base and the alveolar ridge. The vertical distance between the reconstructed segment and the occlusal plane may be excessive, because of the limited height of the fibula barrel (rarely more than 15 mm) compared with the native mandible. This is especially evident when the native mandible is dentate at the unaffected site adjacent to fibula flap. A discrepancy between the vertical height of the grafted bone and that of the native mandible is likely, which causes both aesthetic and functional problems. Insufficient lip support may be related to depressed lower lip and poor chin profile. In implant-borne dental rehabilitation, if the reconstructed alveolar ridge is low, we may get an inadequate crown-to-implant ratio (i.e. long prosthetic teeth) that may result in early implant failure. In cases of high discrepancy, the implants have to support very long prosthetic suprastructures to reach the occlusal plane, with the risk of unfavourable bending moments and implant overloading, which may jeopardize the longevity of the prosthetic restoration [1, 2].

Anesi et al. (2018) demonstrated that osteotomies performed using piezosurgical devices show more advanced stages of bone healing compared with rotary instruments. Moreover, even more powerful devices (output power of 75 W) do not alter the process of bone healing. Generally speaking, we recommend piezosurgical devices for improved bone healing when osteotomies are planned in bone augmentation [3, 4]. In delayed bone augmentation, planning accurate evaluation for previous administration of bisphosphonate or other antiresorptive drug treatment should be made, in order to avoid medication-related osteonecrosis of the jaw (MRONJ) and antiresorptive drug-related osteonecrosis of the jaw (ARONJ) [5].

The use of bone substitutes in fibula flap augmentation is not described in the literature, although new HA/bioactive glass composites have already been tested in animal model [6, 7].

To overcome the high discrepancy between the reconstructed alveolar crest and the native one, some therapeutic options have been introduced: fixation of the fibula at the level of the residual alveolar crest of the healthy side, primary use of the fibula as a double-barrel graft, delayed onlay bone graft on the fibula, later vertical distraction osteogenesis and secondary osteotomies to correct malocclusion after fibula.

The first of these options, fixating the fibula mono-barrel at the level of the residual alveolar ridge of the native mandible, is not recommended, because the lower mandible profile, the angle and the facial contour may be adversely affected.

Other techniques for vertical bone augmentation in fibula flap are now discussed.

Double-Barrel Graft

The double-barrel graft technique consists of placing two fibula fragments positioned parallel and adjacent to each other, like the two barrels of a gun. Fibula's blood supply is sufficient to support multiple osteotomies; therefore it meets the prerequisite for double-barrel technique [8–10].

The advantages of double-barrel fibula technique are as follows: no later operation is needed for vertical augmentation compared with the onlay bone graft and distraction of the fibula; high-quality bone suitable for implant-anchored rehabilitation is obtained [11].

P. F. Nocini (✉) · A. Fior
Division of Oral and Maxillo-Facial Surgery, University Hospital of Verona, Verona, Italy
e-mail: pierfrancesco.nocini@univr.it; andrea.fior@aovr.veneto.it

A. Anesi
Cranio-Maxillo-Facial Surgery Unit, University Hospital of Modena, Modena, Italy
e-mail: alexandre.anesi@unimore.it

G. De Santis et al. (eds.), *Atlas of Mandibular and Maxillary Reconstruction with the Fibula Flap*,
https://doi.org/10.1007/978-3-030-10684-3_7

Limits of double-barrel fibula technique are reached in the case of large mandible defects: the length of the bone segment may not be enough for duplication of the entire reconstructed part. Moreover, this method is technically demanding, with a higher risk of pedicle thrombosis related to pedicle kinking between the two barrels. In some patients the diameter of the fibula is so large that a double-barrel reconstruction occupies the prosthetic space related to upper dentition; damages caused by opposing teeth may occur on the revascularized flap [2].

The specificity of dental implants on double-barrel graft is that they require a bicortical placement (Figs. 1–10) or, if possible, a tricortical placement, which means that the implants should be transfixed through both fragments [15–17].

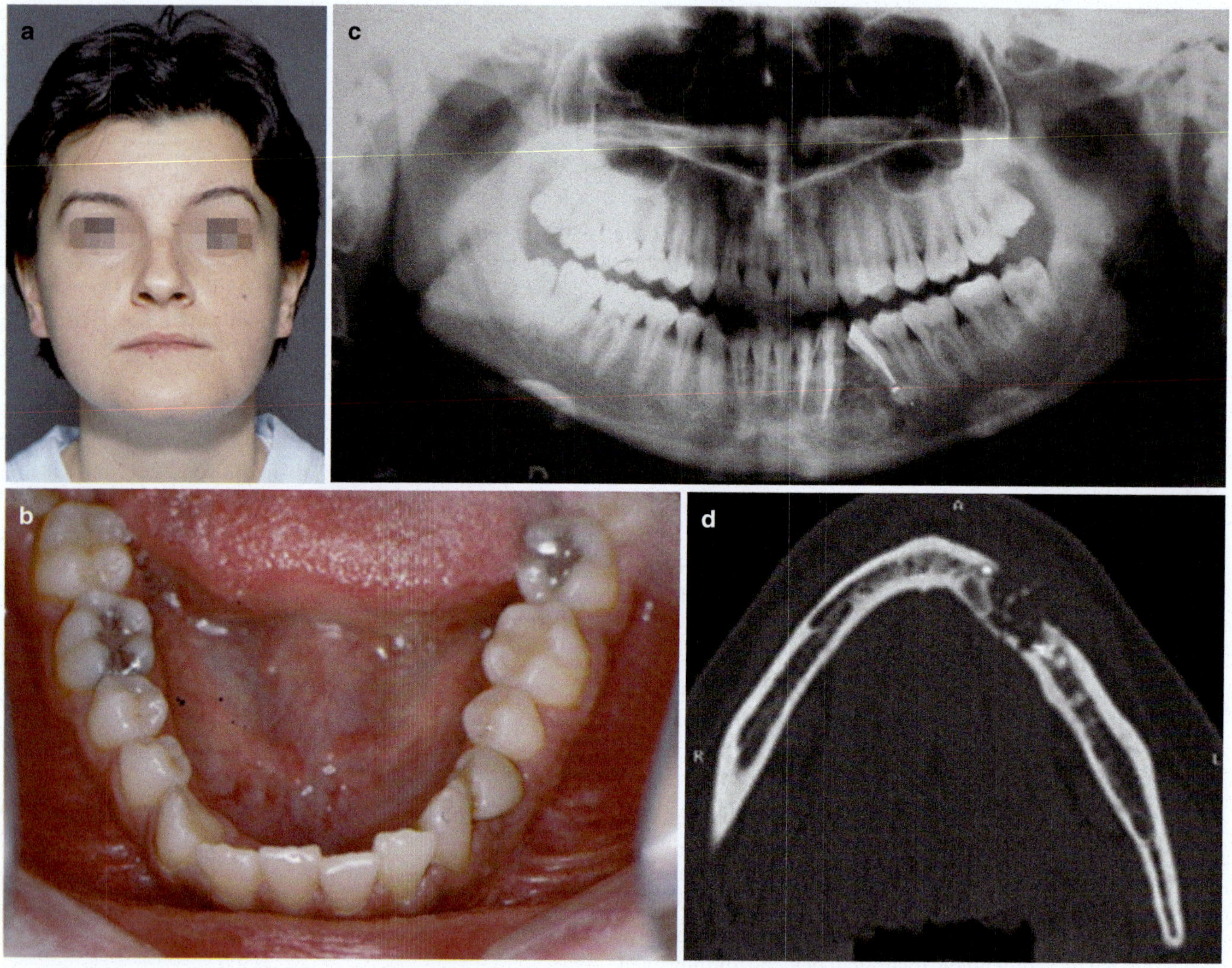

Fig. 1 (**a**) Frontal view of the patient. (**b**) Intraoral view with dystopia of 33 dental element. (**c**) Orthopantomograph. Left mandibular ameloblastoma between 33 and 34 dental elements. (**d**) CT scan shows osteolytic lesion related to ameloblastoma growth [12–14]

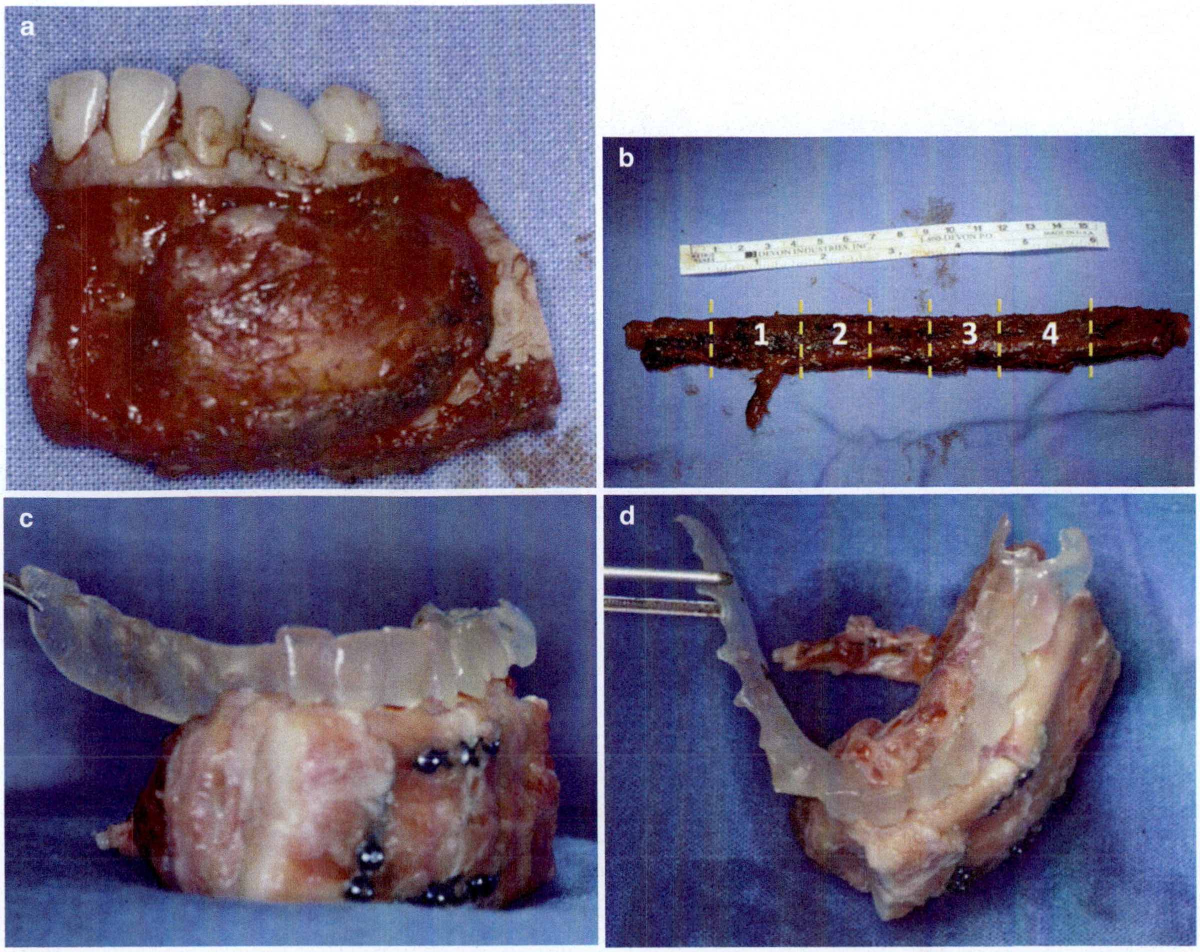

Fig. 2 (**a**) Parasymphyseal segmental mandibulectomy. (**b**) Fibula flap harvested at a side table. Note the marks for six osteotomies to get two bony segments followed by a 3 cm discarded segment and two further segments. (**c** and **d**) Upper and lower barrels are fixed together. Discarding this segment, the periosteal blood supply can safely bridge the two barrels once folded. A dental template guided fibula shaping

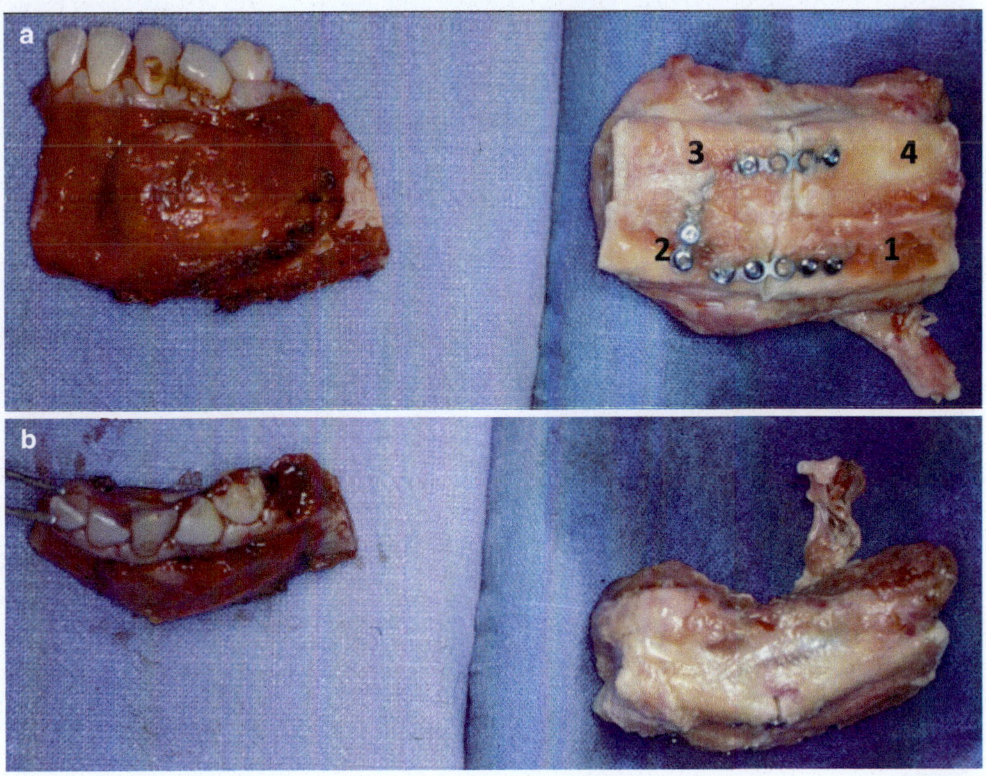

Fig. 3 (**a** and **b**) Good matching between the resected specimen and the contoured fibula flap

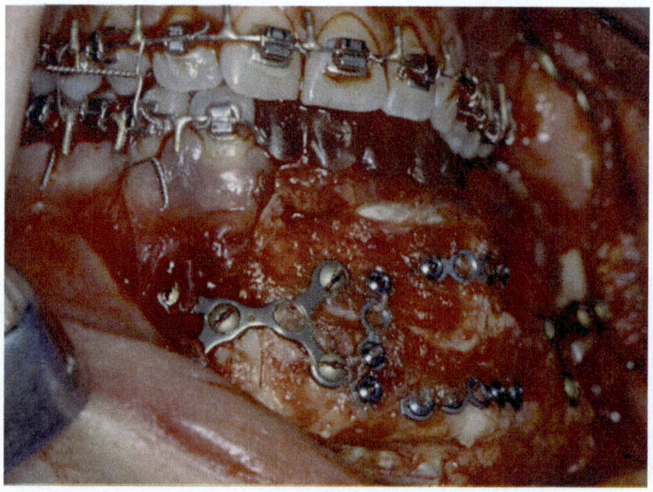

Fig. 4 Fibula flap insetting. Note the accurate positioning and fixation of the flap thanks to rigid intermaxillary fixation and dental template

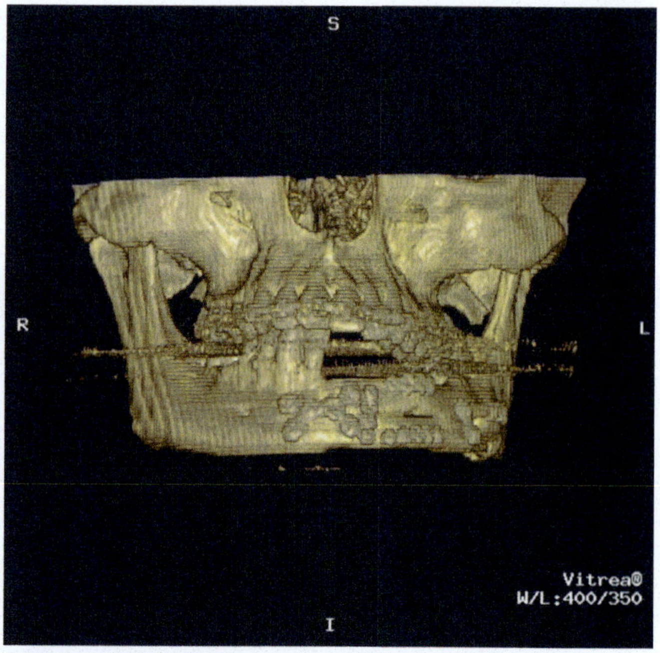

Fig. 5 Postoperative 3D CT scan

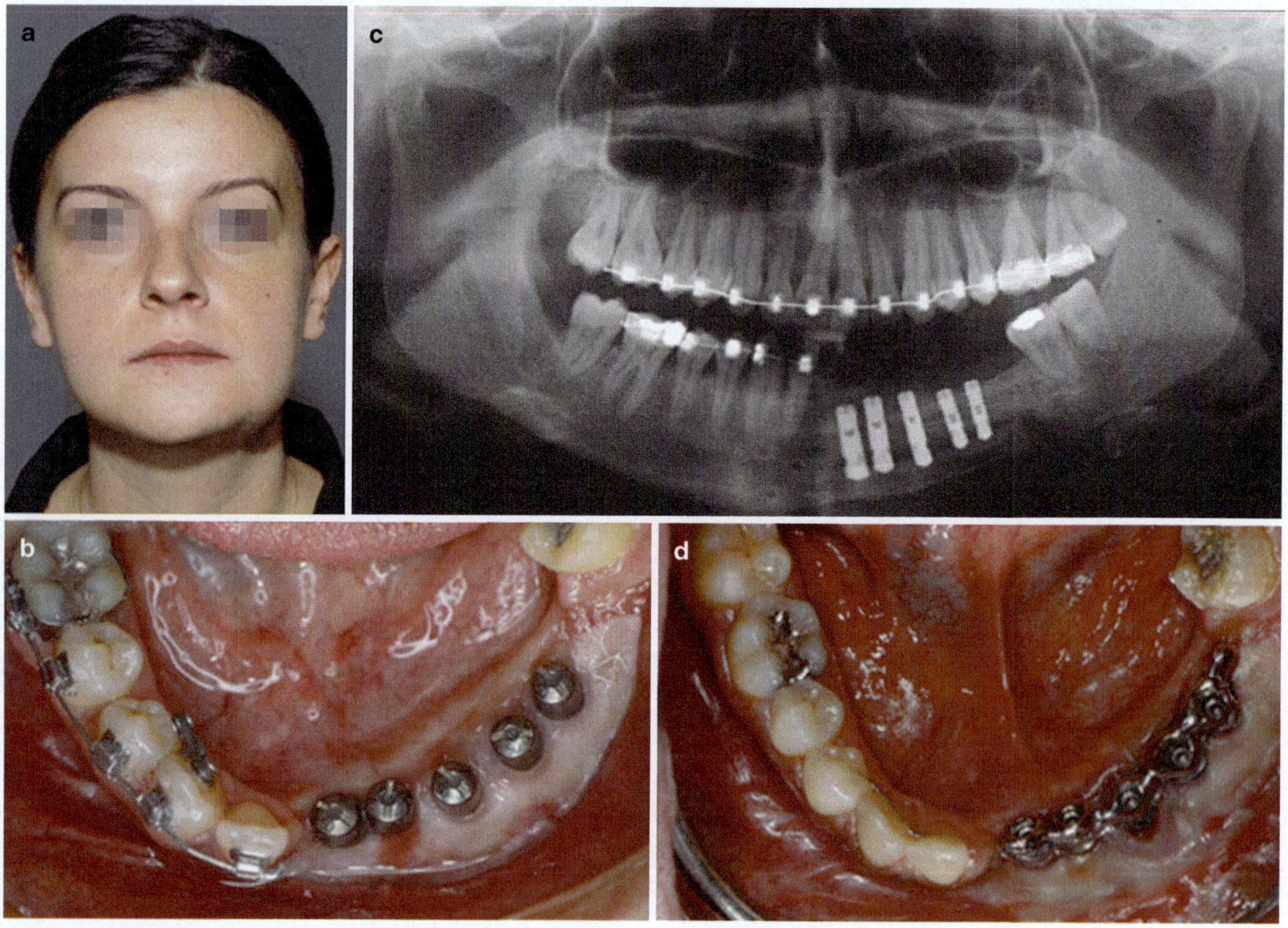

Fig. 6 (**a**) Postoperative frontal view of the patient. (**b**) Peri-implant soft tissue healed. (**c**) Postoperative orthopantomograph with evidence of tricortical placement of endosseous dental implants in fibula flap. (**d**) Occlusal view showing the metalwork in situ on the top of the abutments

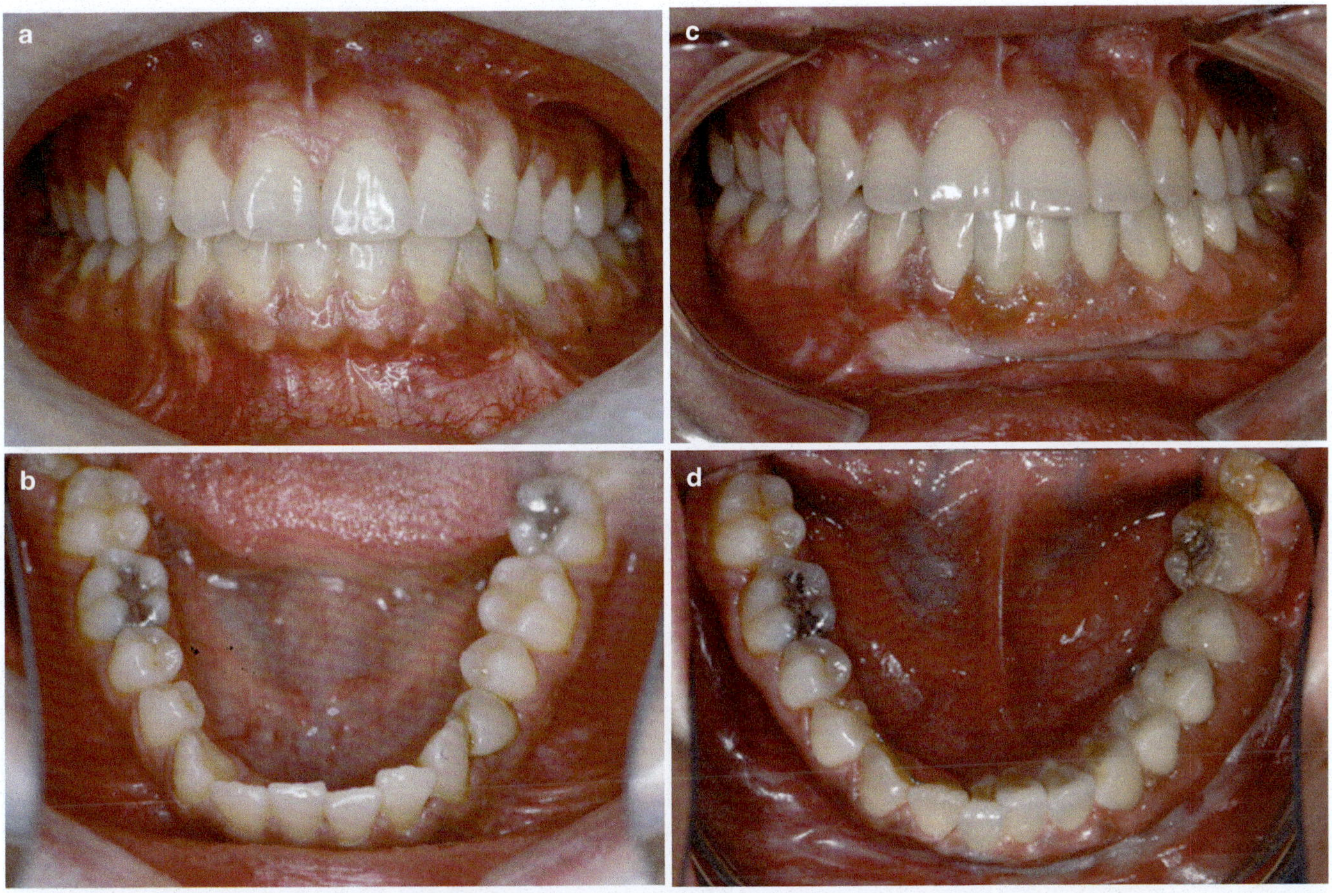

Fig. 7 (**a** and **b**) Comparison between preoperative dental occlusal status and (**c** and **d**) postoperative prosthetic rehabilitation

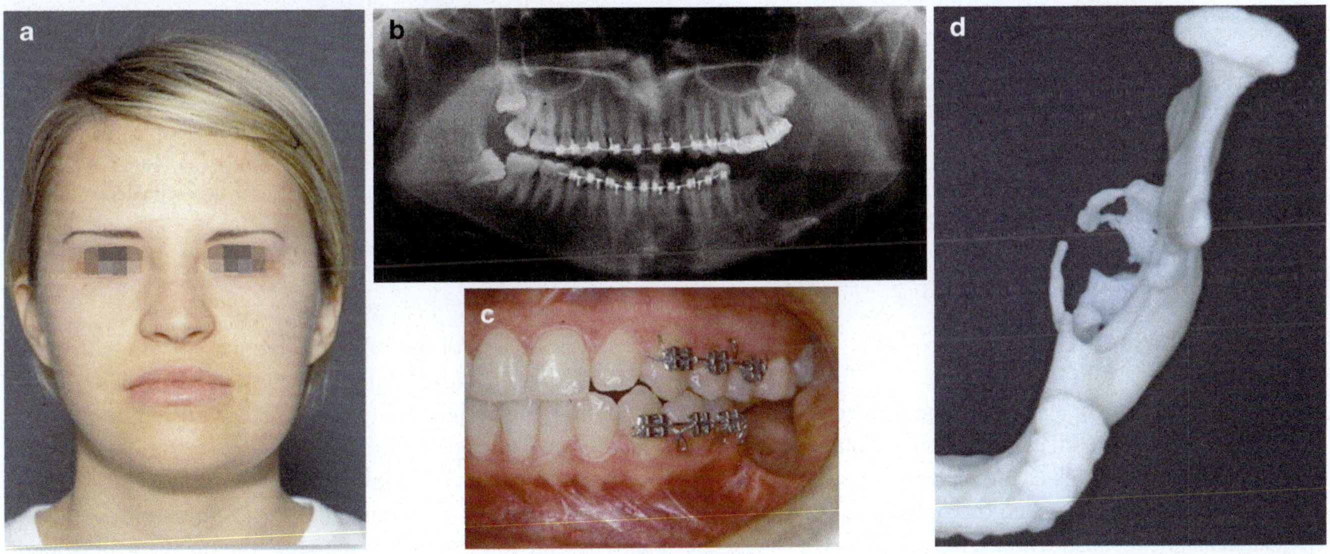

Fig. 8 Left hemimandibular relapse of giant cell granuloma after medical treatment. (**a**) Lower left cheek swelling in a 19-year-old girl. (**b**) Large radiolucency in orthopantomography. (**c**) Intraoral view. (**d**) Stereolithographic model with bony lesion [13, 14]

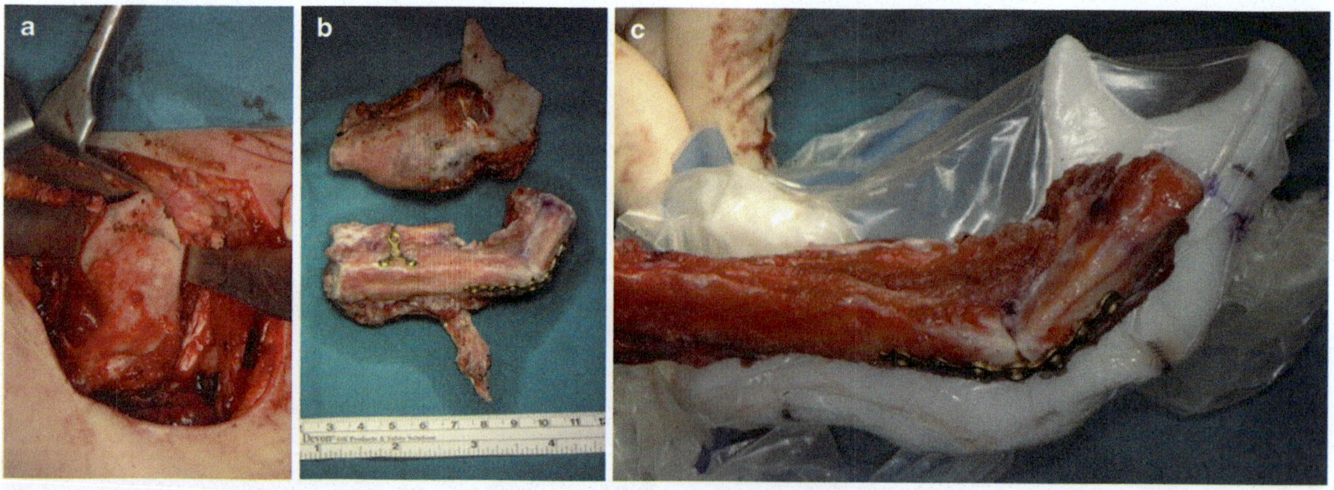

Fig. 9 (**a**) Intraoperative segmental mandibular resection. (**b**) Intraoperative comparison between resected surgical specimen and fibula flap contoured with double-barrelling technique. (**c**) Compare between shaped fibula flap and stereolithographic model

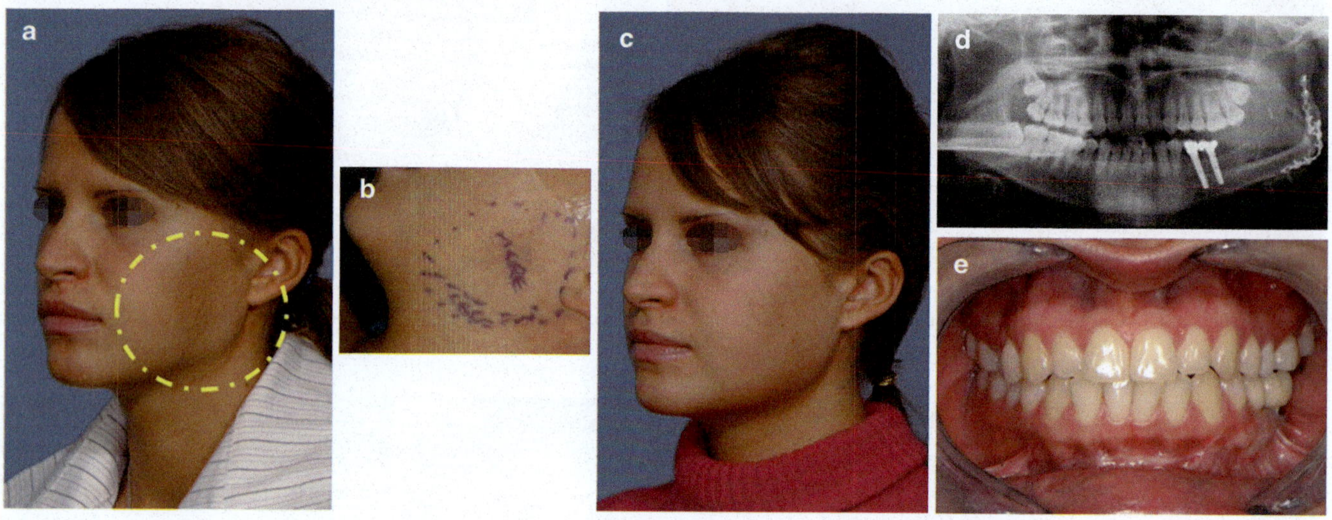

Fig. 10 (**a**) Postoperative ¾ portrait where soft tissue deficit was outlined at the left cheek. (**b**) Intraoperative skin mark for lipofilling procedure. (**c**) ¾ portrait after left cheek lipofilling. (**d**) Postoperative orthopantomograph with evidence of tricortical placement of endosseous dental implants in fibula flap. (**e**) Occlusal view with dental implant-borne prosthetic rehabilitation

Non-vascularized Graft

Delayed autologous onlay iliac bone graft onto the fibula flap to restore the alveolar arch up to the occlusal plane is described [2, 18, 19]. However, this technique is rarely accepted by the patient who has recently undergone a major surgical intervention, such as jaw reconstruction (Figs. 11–16).

Lee and coworkers [2] reported a unique intervention for the basal mandibular bone reconstruction with a standard fibular graft and for the superior alveolar portion with a non-vascularized residual fibular segment and bone chips. Although the bone volume is correctly restored through this technique, delayed healing and infection ratio are higher compared to conventional mono-barrel fibula. Between the non-vascularized graft and the fibula, intervening fibrosis may occur. In oral cancer patients, the need for postoperative irradiation can influence bone resorption and graft viability.

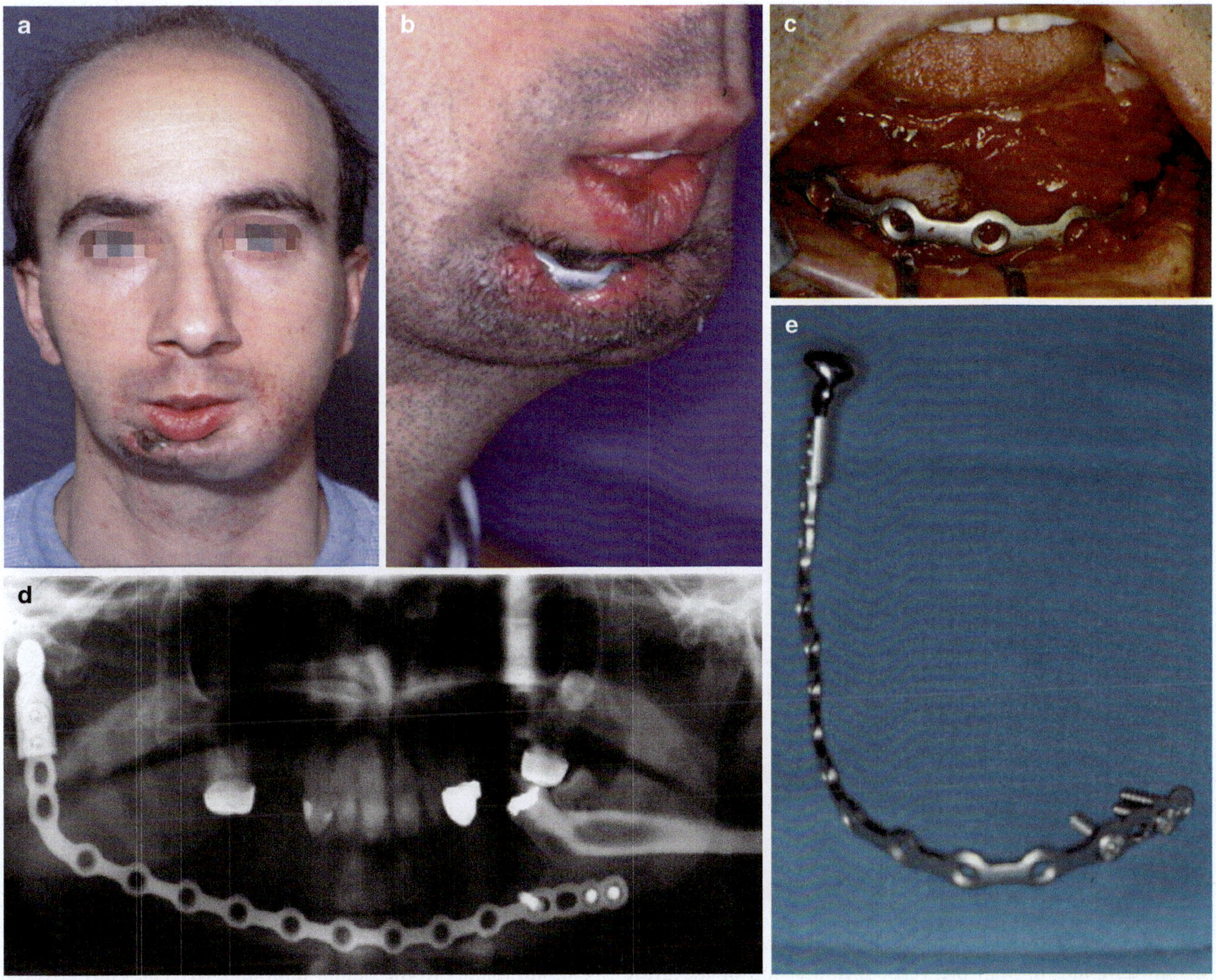

Fig. 11 Wide post-traumatic right hemimandibular defect treated by rib graft and reconstruction titanium plate. (**a** and **b**) Skin exposition of the reconstruction plate. (**c**) Intraoral view of the reconstruction plate and torn skin. (**d**) Orthopantomograph with the reconstruction plate and rib bone resorption. (**e**) The titanium plate after the removal

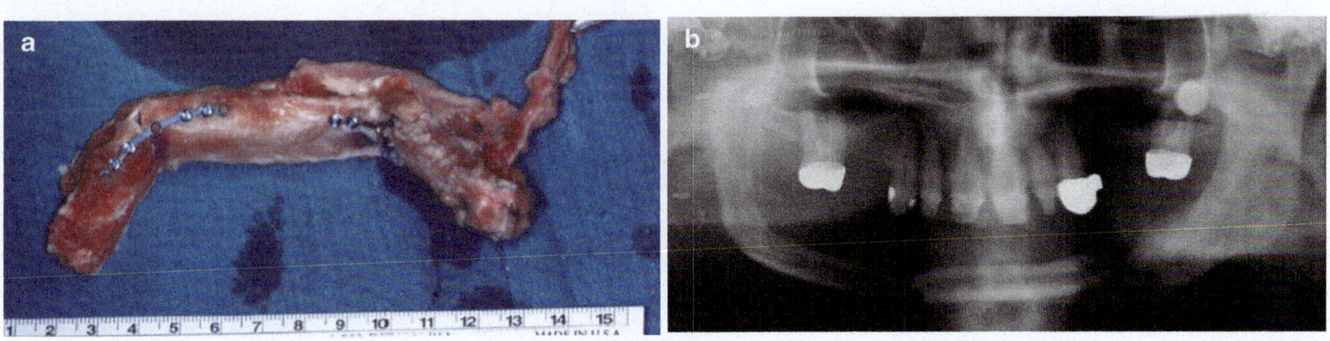

Fig. 12 (**a**) Fibula flap harvested and shaped according to mandibular arch. (**b**) Postoperative orthopantomograph

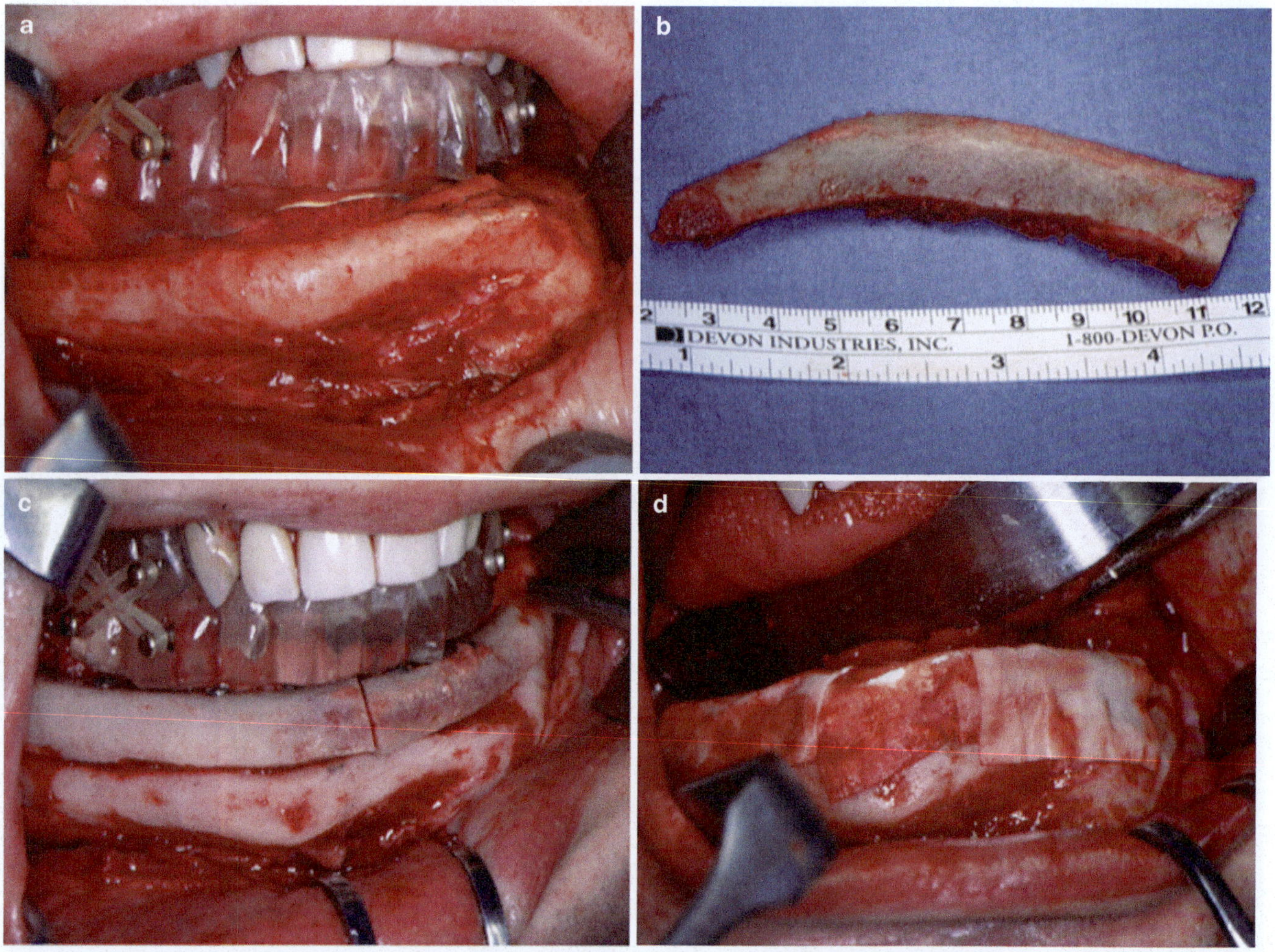

Fig. 13 (**a**) Elastic intermaxillary fixation with positioned dental template to plan the vertical dimension of the graft. (**b**) Large non-revascularized autologous iliac crest graft. (**c**) The graft is accurately positioned and fixed onto the fibula flap thanks to the dental template. (**d**) The graft covered by collagen membranes

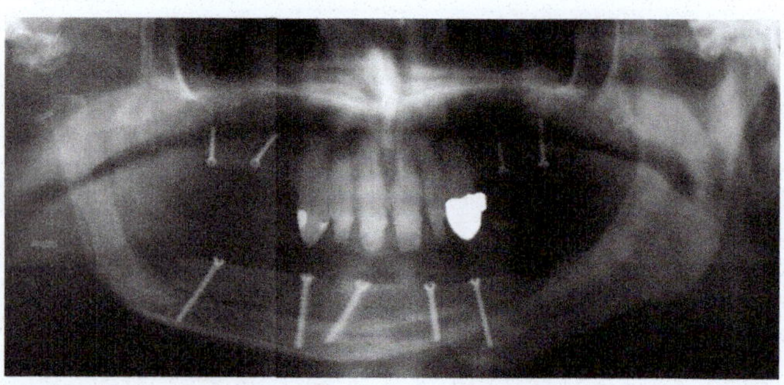

Fig. 14 Postoperative orthopantomograph after vertical bone augmentation

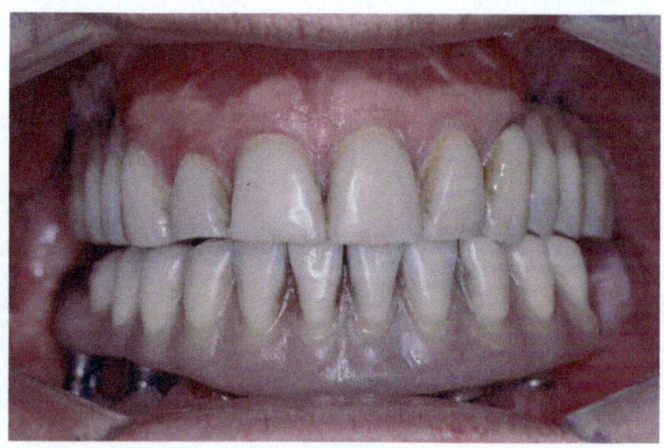

Fig. 15 Implant-borne dental prosthetic rehabilitation

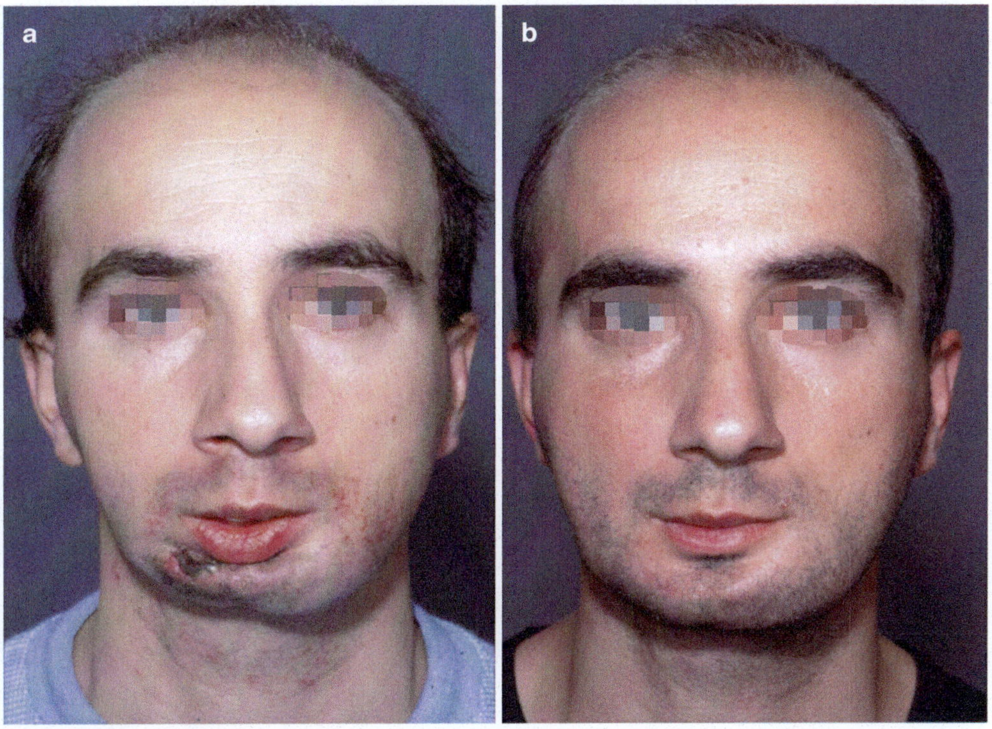

Fig. 16 (**a**) Preoperative and (**b**) postoperative frontal view of the patient

Distraction Osteogenesis

Distraction osteogenesis, performed in cases of vertical resorption of edentulous jaws to improve bone volume for dental implant placement (alveolar distraction), is well described in the scientific literature. The bone quality provided by this technique is good and suitable for endosseous dental implant positioning [20, 21].

From this experience, Nocini et al. [1] reported a case of bone vertical augmentation through distraction osteogenesis after fibula graft (Figs. 17–24).

The guidelines in the literature describe clearly what to do for adequate bone-borne distractor positioning. The risk of damaging the pedicle during horizontal osteotomy should be considered. The lingual periosteal blood supply of the fibula during dissection has to be carefully preserved. If two more distractors have been planned, the two devices are applied parallel to each other to gain precise three-dimensional bone growth. The distraction vector was perpendicular to the major axis of the fibula [1, 17].

After distractor positioning, a latency period lasting 10 days must be maintained. The distraction rate was 0.5 mm per day, and the consolidation period lasted 3 months [1, 22].

Ultrasound scanning provides a non-invasive follow-up of bone growth inside the distracted area [1].

Intraoral distractor is related to aggravated oral hygiene, and an increased risk of recurrent soft tissue infection is reported. Distraction osteogenesis presents some limitations when the fibula shaft is particularly thin; complicated wound healing may occur in irradiated patients [2, 18, 19].

The reported stable increase in vertical bone height with distraction osteogenesis after the fibula flap is from 11 to 15 mm [22].

The success of dental implants in fibula free flap ranges from 93.1% with a mean follow-up of 50.2 months to 96.1% after 2 years [15]. Peri-implant bone resorption can occur if no keratinized oral mucosa is present. The maintenance of good oral hygiene is essential in rehabilitation after reconstruction with free fibula flap.

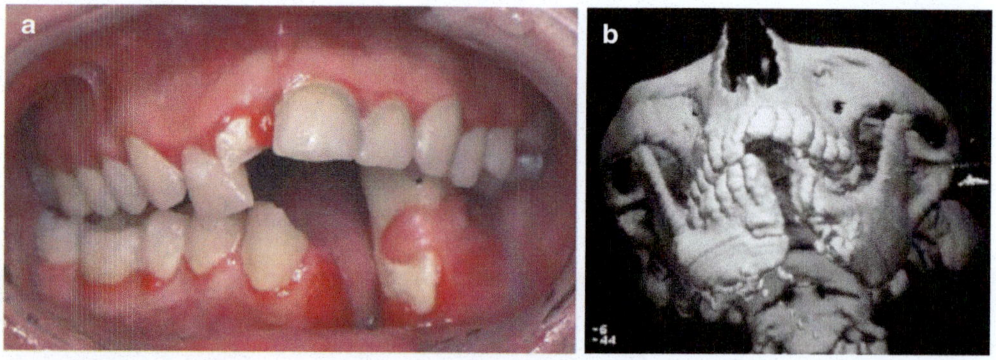

Fig. 17 (**a**) Intraoral view of gunshot post-traumatic mandibular parasymphyseal defect. (**b**) CT 3D reconstruction

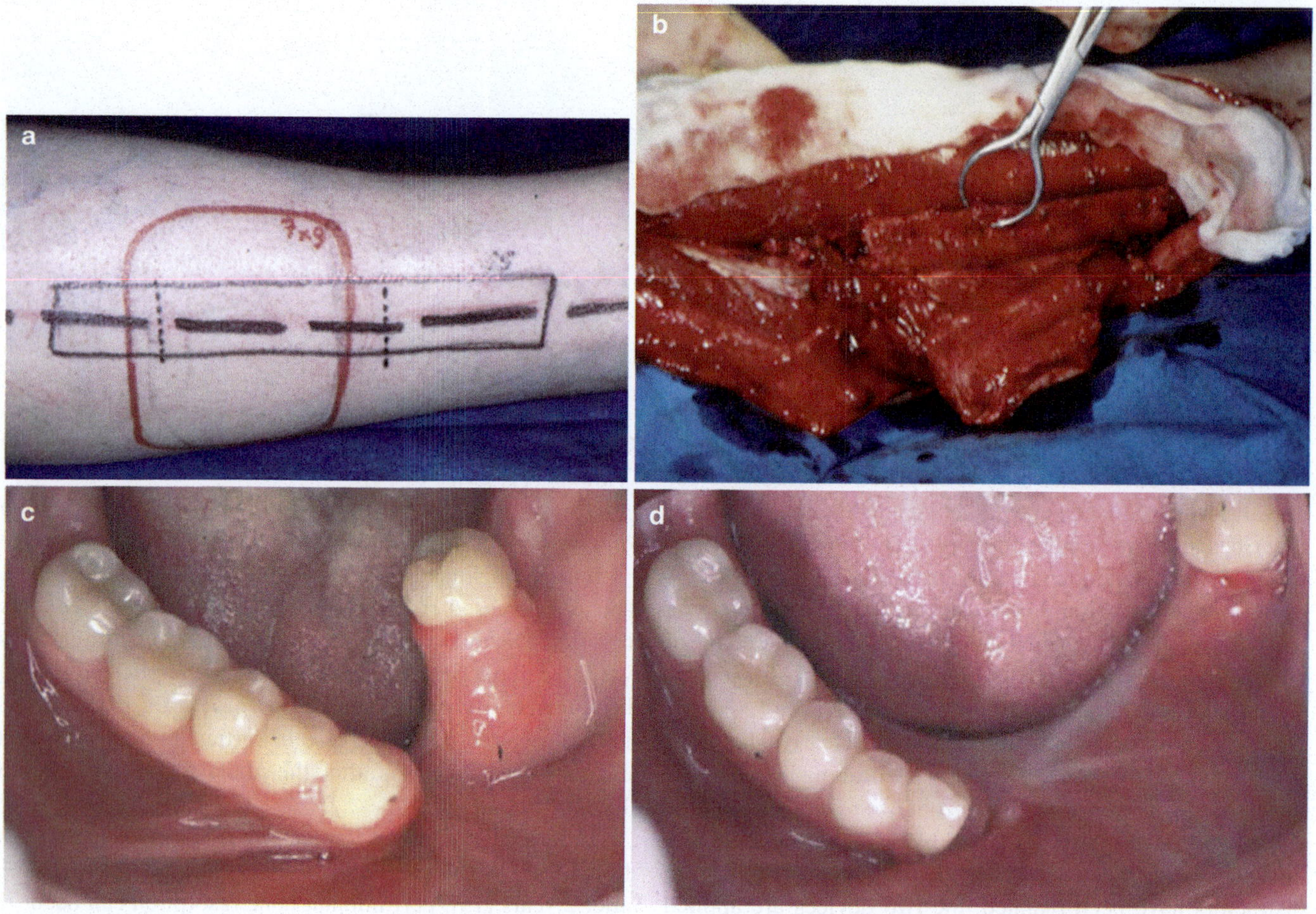

Fig. 18 (**a**) Preoperative drawing before fibula flap harvesting. (**b**) Fibula flap harvested. (**c** and **d**) Comparison between dental inferior arch before and after mandibular reconstruction

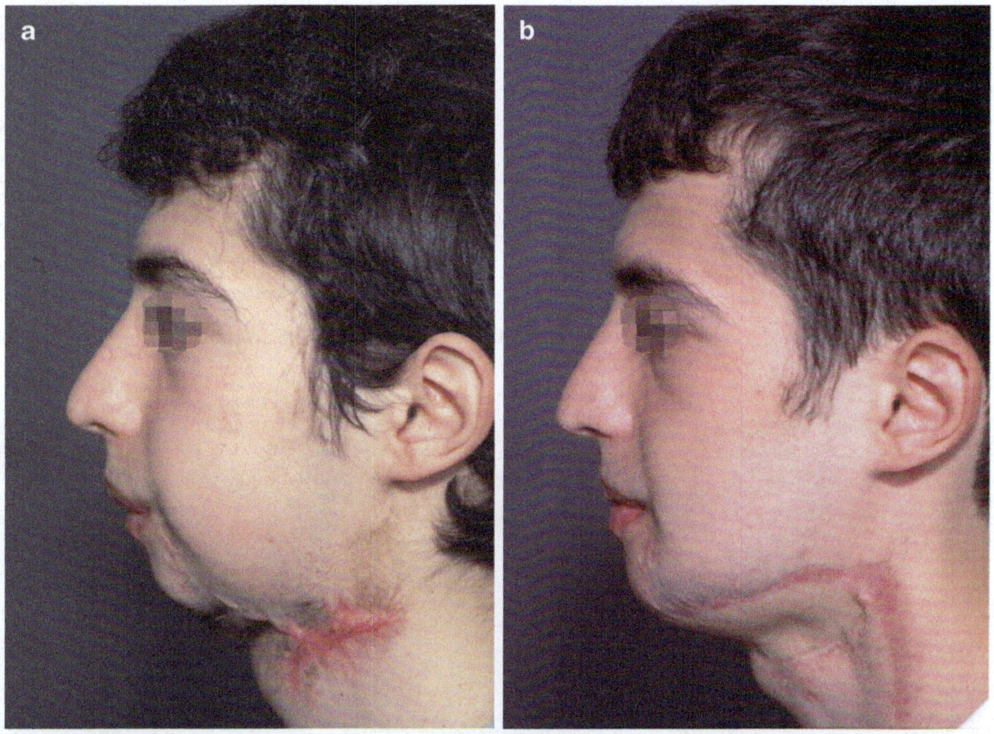

Fig. 19 (**a**) Preoperative and (**b**) postoperative profile of patient in Figs. 17 and 18

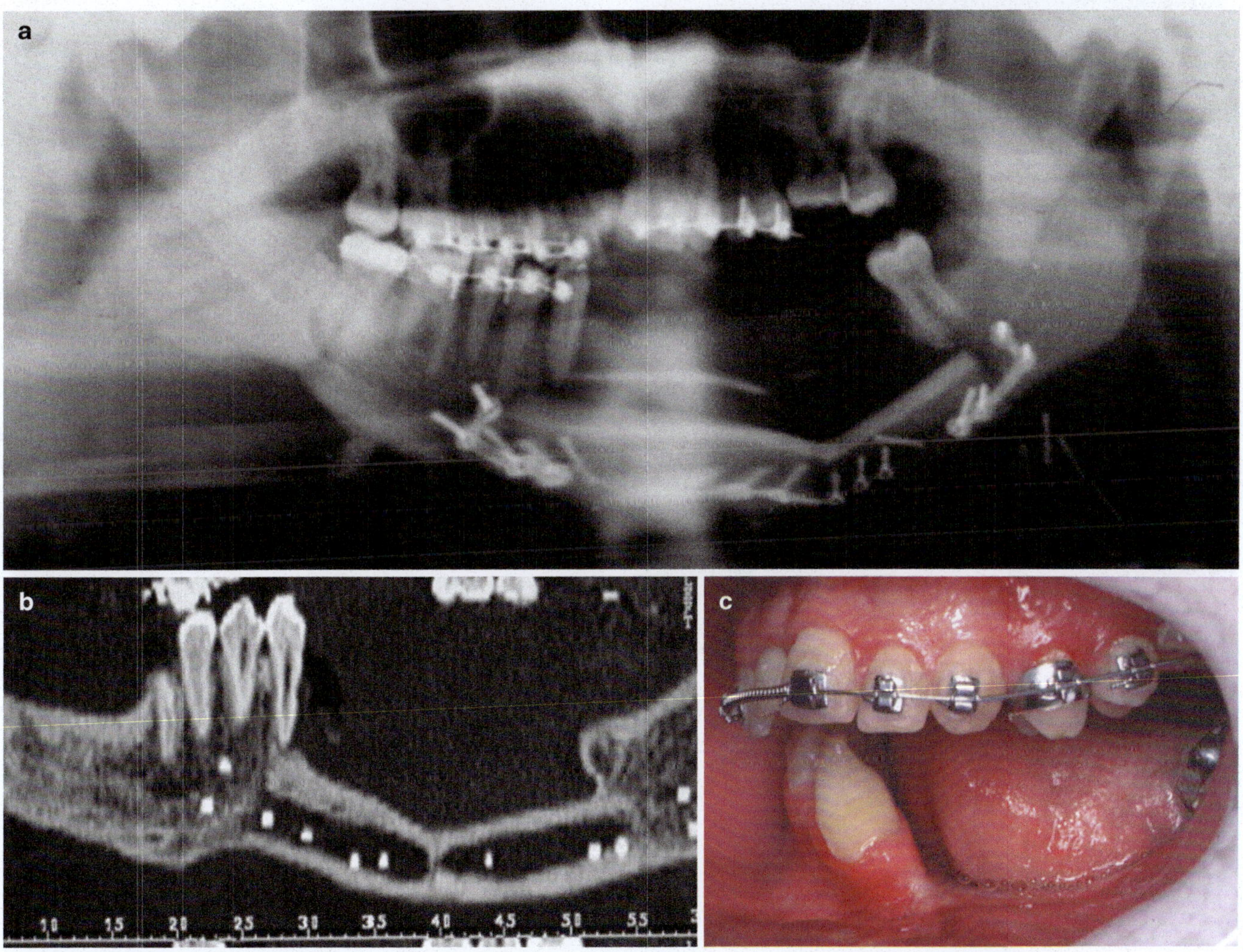

Fig. 20 (**a–c**) Vertical discrepancy in height after fibula flap was demonstrated both in orthopantomograph and CT and intraoral examination

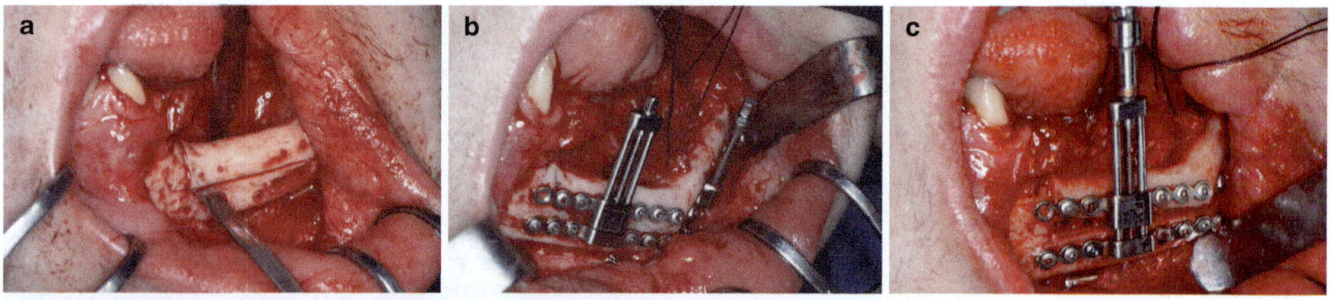

Fig. 21 (**a**) Fibula axial osteotomy was performed. (**b** and **c**) Two intraoral distractors for osteogenesis were in parallel positioned

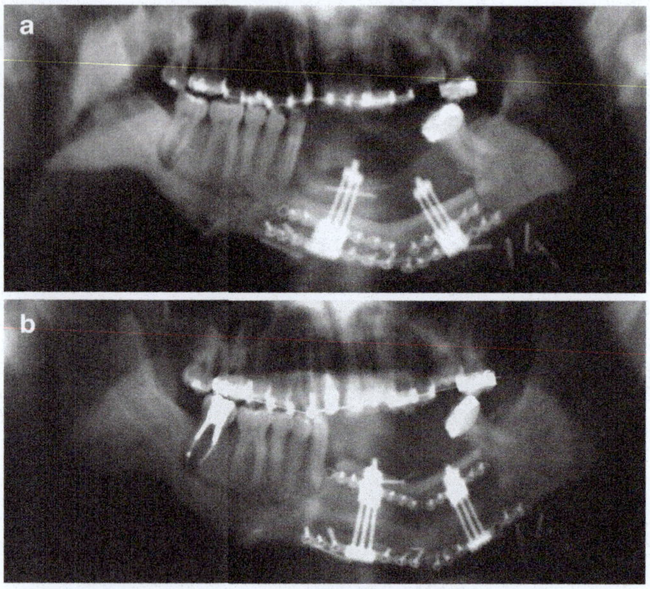

Fig. 22 (**a**) Postoperative orthopantomograph (**a**) at the beginning and (**b**) at the end of distraction osteogenesis

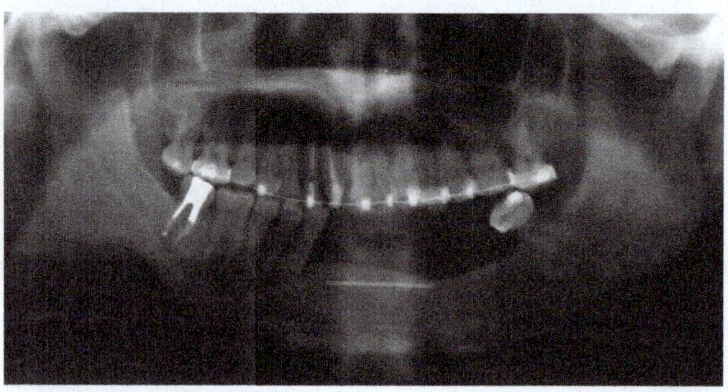

Fig. 23 Postoperative orthopantomograph with an adequate height of left mandibular body

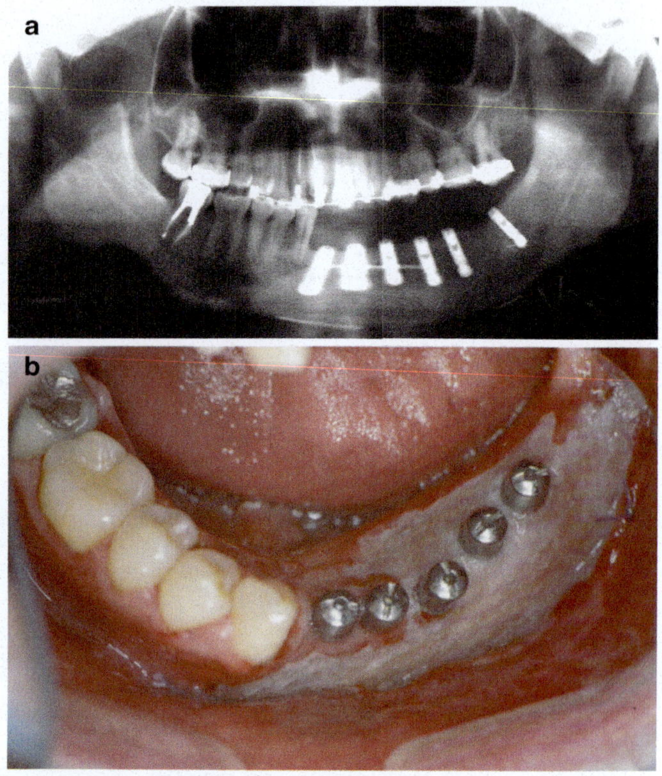

Fig. 24 (**a**) Dental endosseous implant were positioned. (**b**) Healed soft tissue peri-implant tissues

References

1. Nocini PF, Wangerin K, Albanese M, Kretschmer W, Cortelazzi R. Vertical distraction of a free vascularized fibula flap in a reconstructed hemimandible: case report. J Craniomaxillofac Surg. 2000;28:20–4.
2. Lee JH, Kim MJ, Choi WS, Yoon PY, Ahn KM, Myung H, et al. Concomitant reconstruction of mandibular basal and alveolar bone with a free fibular flap. Int J Oral Maxillofac Surg. 2004;33:150–6.
3. Anesi A, Ferretti M, Cavani F, Salvatori R, Bianchi M, Russo A, Chiarini L, Palumbo C. Structural and ultrastructural analyses of bone regeneration in rabbit cranial osteotomy: Piezosurgery versus traditional osteotomes. J Craniomaxillofac Surg. 2018;46(1):107–18. https://doi.org/10.1016/j.jcms.2017.10.004. Epub 2017 Oct 12
4. Turra M, Bertossi D, Bissolotti G, Anesi A, Chiarini L, Nocini PF. 0.095 Genioplasty with piezosurgery. J Craniomaxillofac Surg. 2008;36(Supp.1):S24. https://doi.org/10.1016/S1010-5182(08)71219-8.
5. Pozzi S, Anesi A, Generali L, Bari A, Consolo U, Chiarini L. Bisphosphonate-related osteonecrosis of the jaw (BRONJ). In: Tsesis I, editor. Complications in endodontic surgery: prevention, identification and management. 1st ed. New York: Springer-Verlag Berlin Heidelberg; 2014. p. 153–65. https://doi.org/10.1007/978-3-642-54218-3.. ISBN 978-3-642-54217-6; ISBN 978-3-642-54218-3 (eBook).
6. Bellucci D, Anesi A, Salvatori R, Chiarini L, Cannillo V. A comparative in vivo evaluation of bioactive glasses and bioactive glass-based composites for bone tissue repair. Mater Sci Eng C. 2017;79:286–95.
7. Bellucci D, Sola A, Salvatori R, Anesi A, Chiarini L, Cannillo V. Role of magnesium oxide and strontium oxide as modifiers in silicate-based bioactive glasses: effects on thermal behaviour, mechanical properties and in-vitro bioactivity. Korean J Couns Psychother. 2017;72:566–75.
8. Jones NF, Swartz WM, Mears DC, Jupiter JB, Grossman A. The “double barrel” free vascularized fibular bone graft. Plast Reconstr Surg. 1988;81:378–85.
9. Horiuchi K, Hattori A, Inada I, Kamibayashi T, Sugimura M, Yajima H, et al. Mandibular reconstruction using the double barrel fibular graft. Microsurgery. 1995;16(7):450 4.
10. Bähr W, Stoll P, Wächter R. Use of the “double barrel” free vascularized fibula in mandibular reconstruction. J Oral Maxillofac Surg. 1998;56(1):38–44.
11. He Y, Zhang ZY, Zhu HG, Wu YQ, Fu HH. Double-barrel fibula vascularized free flap with dental rehabilitation for mandibular reconstruction. J Oral Maxillofac Surg. 2011;69(10):2663–9. Erratum in: J Oral Maxillofac Surg. 2012;70(1):251.
12. Anesi A, Bissolotti G, Toller N, Corrocher G, Chiarini L, Nocini PF. Ameloblastic flbroma in a 6-year-old child: case report. J Craniomaxillofac Surg. 2008;36(Supp.1):S81. https://doi.org/10.1016/S1010-5182(08)71446-X.
13. Anesi A. An aggressive ameloblastic fibroma in a 9-year-old child treated with buccal fat graft. J Cranio-Maxillary Dis. 2013;2:85–6. ISSN: 2278-9588
14. Anesi A, Albanese M, Gerosa R, Corrocher G, Gambarini G, Nocini PF. Mandibular ameloblastic fibroma in 6-years-old girl: a case report. Minerva Stomatol. 2008;57(10):549–55. English, Italian
15. Chiapasco M, Biglioli F, Autelitano L, Romeo E, Brusati R. Clinical outcome of dental implants placed in fibula-free flaps used for the reconstruction of maxillo-mandibular defects following ablation for tumors or osteoradionecrosis. Clin Oral Implants Res. 2006;17(2):220–8.
16. Smolka K, Kraehenbuehl M, Eggensperger N, Hallermann W, Thoren H, Iizuka T, et al. Fibula free flap reconstruction of the mandible in cancer patients: evaluation of a combined surgical and prosthodontic treatment concept. Oral Oncol. 2008;44(6):571–81.
17. Chang YM, Wallace CG, Tsai CY, Shen YF, Hsu YM, Wei FC. Dental implant outcome after primary implantation into double-barreled fibula osteoseptocutaneous free flap-reconstructed mandible. Plast Reconstr Surg. 2011;128(6):1220–8.
18. Hayter JP, Cawood JI. Oral rehabilitation with endosteal implants and free flaps. Int J Oral Maxillofac Surg. 1996;25:3–12.
19. Hakim SG, Kimmerle H, Trenkle T, Sieg P, Jacobsen HC. Masticatory rehabilitation following upper and lower jaw reconstruction using vascularised free fibula flap and enossal implants-19 years of experience with a comprehensive concept. Clin Oral Investig. 2015;19(2):525–34.
20. Chiapasco M, Brusati R, Galioto S. Distraction osteogenesis of a fibular revascularized flap for improvement of oral implant positioning in a tumor patient: a case report. J Oral Maxillofac Surg. 2000;58:1434–40.
21. Chin M, Toth BA. Distraction osteogenesis in maxillofacial surgery using internal devices: review of five cases. J Oral Maxillofac Surg. 1996;54:45–53.
22. Levin L, Carrasco L, Kazemi A, Chalian A. Enhancement of the fibula free flap by alveolar distraction for dental implant restoration: report of a case. Facial Plast Surg. 2003;19:87–94.

Part IV

Evolution in Concepts

Evolution in Indication

Alexandre Anesi, Sara Negrello, and Luigi Chiarini

Since the introduction of reconstructive technique using the fibula flap, the indications for use of this technique have evolved.

The primary indications for fibular flap have been reconstructions of extended bone defects in the extremities using a posterior approach for flap harvesting. The first fibular flap was performed by Taylor and coworkers, who used a vascularized myosseous segment of the fibula for treatment of a post-traumatic defect of the tibia in 1975 [1].

The fibula graft may provide skin islands, up to 25 cm and 14 cm wide, suitable for reconstruction of associated soft tissue defects.

Chen and Yan were the first to describe the osteocutaneous fibula flap in 1983, following the proposal of Gilbert to use a lateral approach for harvesting the bone flap, which was easier to perform and allowed for visualization of the cutaneous branches of the peroneal artery [2]. The dual endosteal and periosteal blood supply ensures bony viability despite multiple osteotomies.

Hidalgo in 1989 described the first lower jaw reconstruction with a fibular flap, using osteotomies to mimic the shape of the mandible after oncological or traumatic defects [3].

At the beginning of the 1990s, many surgeons were skeptical and hesitant about using the osteocutaneous flap owing to reports that the skin had poor vascular reliability. Experience and a better understanding of the vascular anatomy have improved the viability of the skin paddle.

Multiple skin islands can be harvested with the fibula graft providing an osteomyocutaneous flap, including those based on septocutaneous as well as on musculocutaneous peroneal perforators [4].

The most reliable septocutaneous perforators are located in the middle and distal third of the fibula [5].

Most recently, a second skin island based on proximal perforators off the peroneal artery has been discovered [6].

This graft thus provides convenient tissue for simultaneous reconstruction of bony and soft tissue defects inside as well as outside the oral cavity, bringing viable tissue to a mostly irradiated and contaminated field, with the lowest complication rate among osteocutaneous flaps [7, 8].

Many authors contributed to optimization of the technique by using the soleus muscle connected to motor branches at the recipient site to restore the motor function or by using the sural cutaneous nerve together with a skin island for restoring sensation [9, 10].

To overcome the limited height of the fibula, in 1988 Jones et al. described a modified flap called the double-barrel flap. With this technique, the thickness of the bony portion of the flap can be doubled, and it is normally used in mandibular reconstruction to obtain a flap size equal to the native mandible [11].

Flap combinations were performed by anastomosing a second free flap to the distal peroneal artery and vein, which do not significantly reduce in caliber and thus can also serve at the recipient site [12].

The use of free vascularized fibula has become the gold standard for mandibular and maxillary extensive defects.

Standard indications include bone discontinuity greater than 4–6 cm, with or without any vascular impairment, for any mandibular or maxillary defects [13, 14].

In maxillary defects, regardless of the type of classification we use, we have to consider the extension of the palato-alveolar defect, the conditions of the orbital floor, and whether the *exenteratio orbitae* is needed.

According to Cordeiro's classification, our clinic is able to use fibula flaps for reconstruction of maxilla defect up to type III (A and B) based on the preoperative evaluation of the defect.

The free fibula flap can be shaped (1) to achieve the main reconstructive goals in complex maxillary defects, such as giving support to the orbital contents (Figs. 1–3); (2) to

A. Anesi (✉) · S. Negrello · L. Chiarini
Cranio-Maxillo-Facial Surgery Unit, University Hospital of Modena, Modena, Italy
e-mail: alexandre.anesi@unimore.it; luigi.chiarini@unimore.it

G. De Santis et al. (eds.), *Atlas of Mandibular and Maxillary Reconstruction with the Fibula Flap*,
https://doi.org/10.1007/978-3-030-10684-3_8

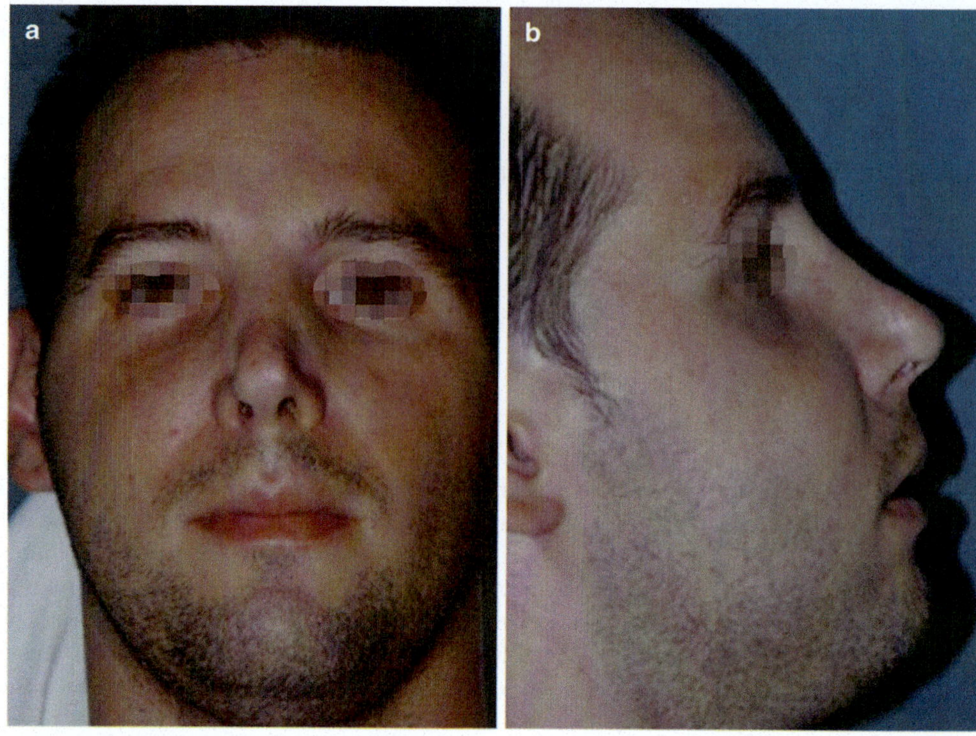

Fig. 1 (**a** and **b**) Frontal and lateral view of patient, note malar prominence due to bulky ameloblastoma of right maxillary bone

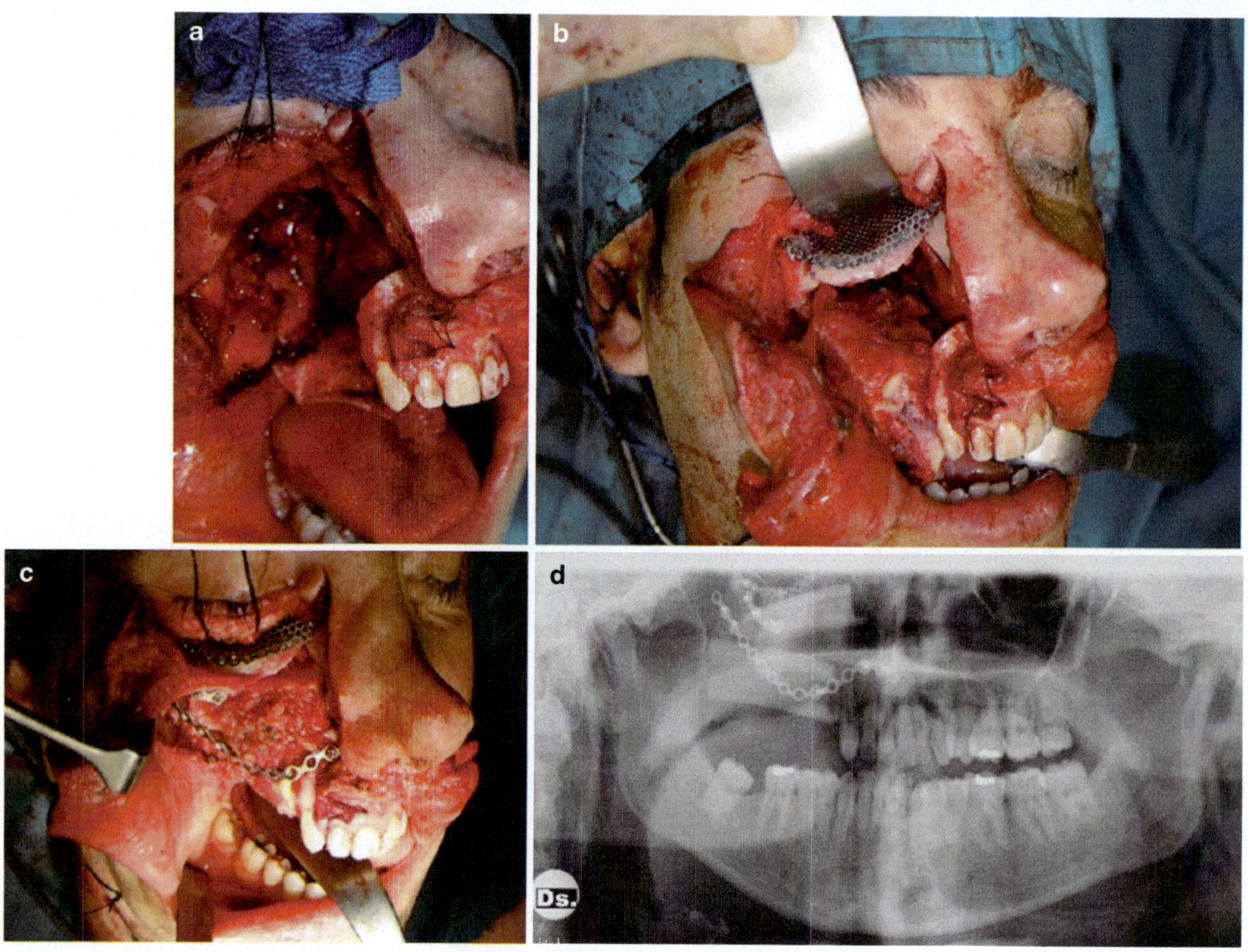

Fig. 2 (**a**) Intraoperative midface defect following extirpation removal of right maxillary ameloblastoma [15, 16] (defect type IIIA, according to Cordeiro's classification). (**b**) Orbital floor reconstruction with titanium mesh. (**c**) Insetting of fibula segments to restore three-dimensional midface volume. Pay attention to the orientation of the bone segments that allows the subsequent dental rehabilitation. (**d**) Postoperative panoramic radiograph (panorex) demonstrates position and fixation of bone segments

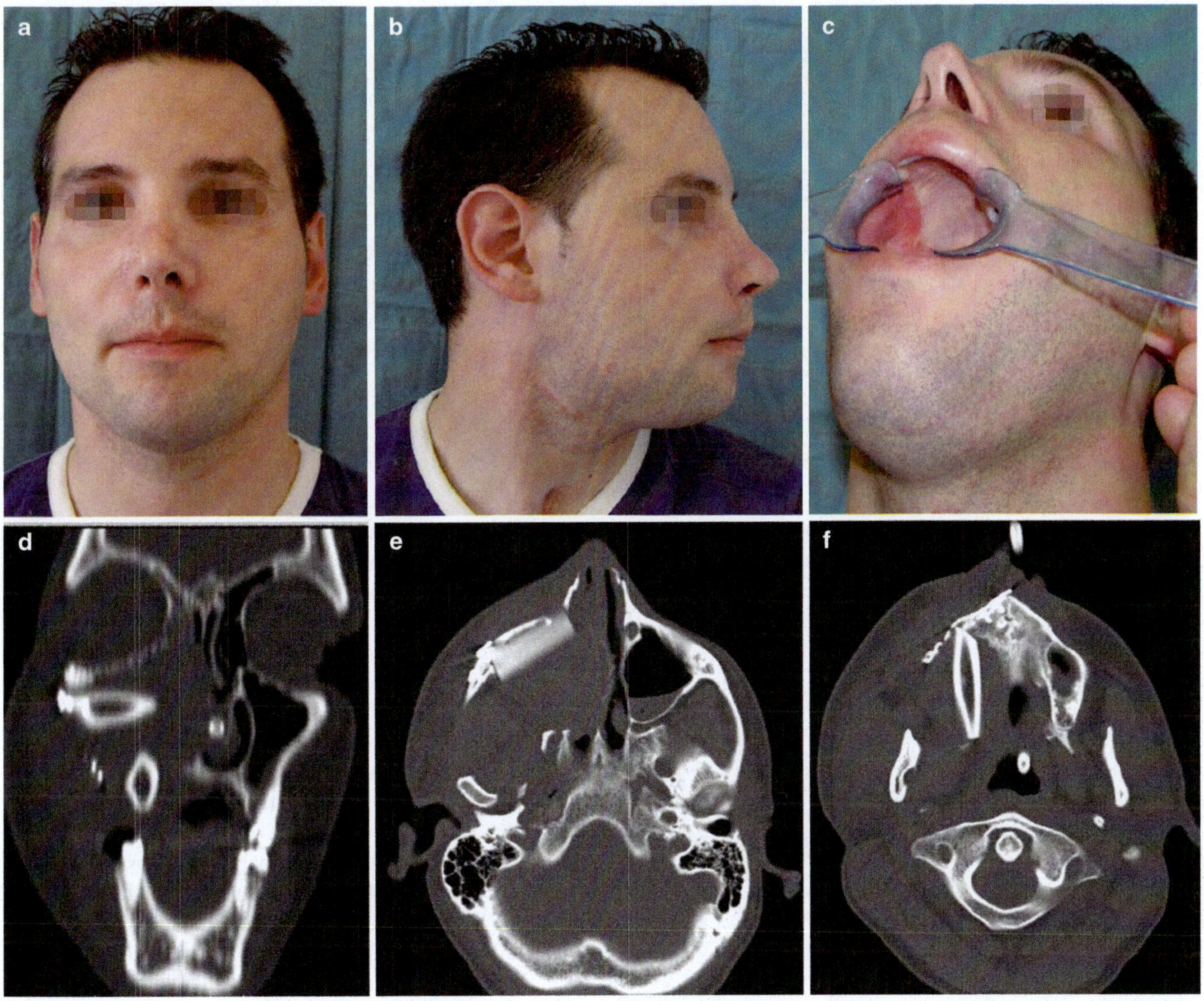

Fig. 3 (**a** and **b**) One-year posttreatment frontal view of the patient after reconstruction. (**c**) Intraoral view. Note the mucosalized palatal surface. (**d**) Coronal CT scan of the patient showing orbital floor reconstruction. (**e** and **f**) Axial Tc scan showing maxillary bone reconstruction

obliterate communication between the mouth, nose, nasopharynx, and anterior cranial base; (3) to reconstruct the palatal and alveolar crest to plan a dental rehabilitation; and (4) to provide enough tissue volume to achieve facial symmetry, thanks to the use of osteo/osteocutaneous/osteomyocutaneous flaps (principle of "like with like reconstruction") [17–19].

Indications for mandibular or maxillary reconstruction are diverse and include oncologic resections (for either benign or malignant tumor), traumatic injuries, congenital defects, osteomyelitis, osteoradionecrosis, and large vascular malformation of the head and neck (Figs. 4–11) [8, 21].

An unusual indication is the reconstruction of temporomandibular joint, which utilizes the ability of the fibula flap to vascularize adjacent segments as cartilage grafts or by suturing the flap to the fibrocartilaginous disk [22]. Certain defects still present difficulties in rehabilitative reconstruction, as the temporomandibular joint does one such site. The condylar head of the mandible is separated from the glenoid fossa by a cartilaginous disk. Disruption of the disk can lead to chronic pain, trismus, and joint instability. Disruption of the condylar head results in incapacitating joint problems (*see* Figs. 6–8 of chapter "Mandible: Lateral, Hemimandibular, Anterior", and Fig. 3 of chapter "Secondary Procedures and Refinements") [23].

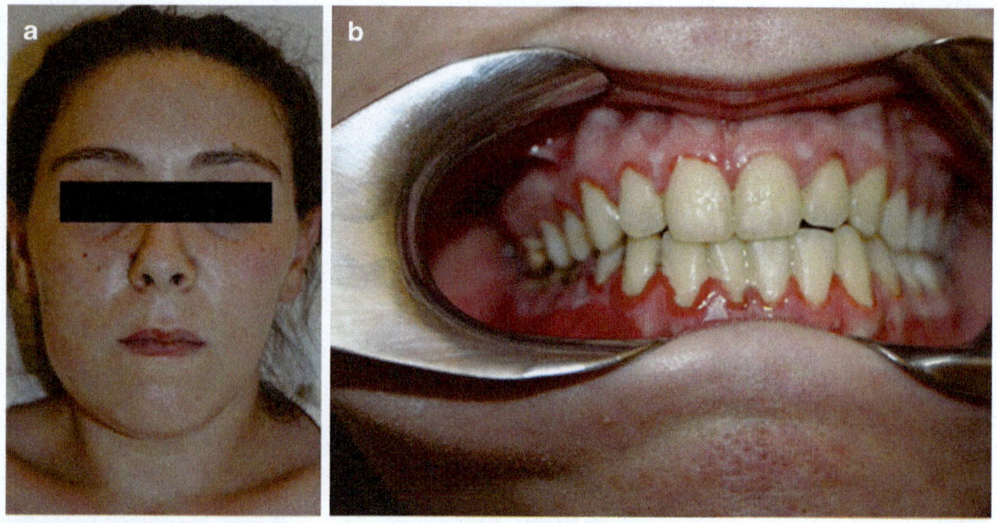

Fig. 4 (**a**) 22-year-old patient preoperative frontal view. Patient presented facial asymmetry with increased size of the lower facial third on the right side due to a mandibular intraosseous arteriovenous malformation. (**b**) Intraoral view showing gingival bleeding and an ecchymotic area extending from the incisive to the retromolar area

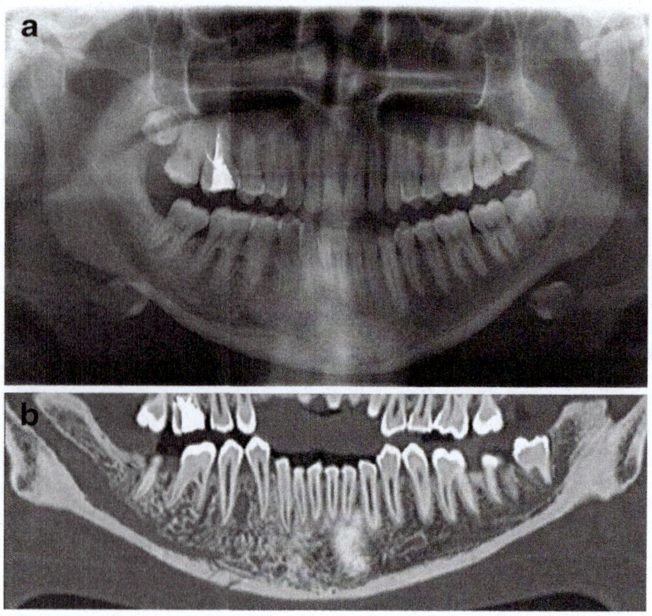

Fig. 5 (**a**) Extensive radiolucency in the right mandible in orthopantomograph. (**b**) Coronal CT scan reconstruction: abnormal enlargement of the right alveolar canal with integral cortical bone

Fibula flap segmentation with piezosurgery is in our opinion more suitable compared to traditional cutting methods, because it improves the intraoperative safety of the procedure, with minimal periosteal elevation [24–27]. We also proved that osteotomies performed using piezosurgical devices show more advanced stages of bone healing compared with rotary instruments. Vertical jaw augmentation mainly involves the lower jaw and to a lesser extent the upper jaws bilaterally. Vertical bone augmentation can be obtained by the "double-barreled technique" or with intraoral bone distraction, in order to offer height to allow placement of dental implants [11]. The "double-barreling" of the fibula enables rapid osseointegrated dental implantation, obtaining better results and lower complication rates compared to vertical distraction devices [17].

Actually, after the development of harvesting and fixation technique, surgeons have extended fibula flap indications to more limited bone defects.

Further indications include:

- Dentoalveolar defects without bone discontinuity.
- Bone discontinuity less than 6 cm.
- Vertical jaws augmentation.

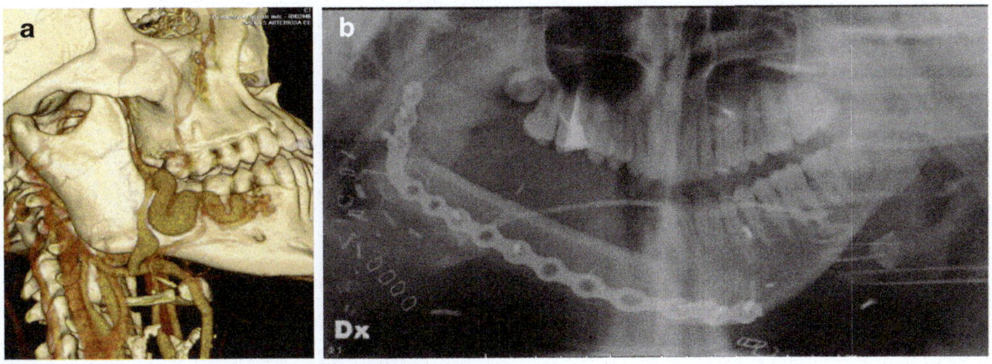

Fig. 6 (**a**) Three-dimensional computed tomography with contrast medium, showing an extensive highly vascularized lesion involving the right side of the mandible and right submandibular region. (**b**) Postoperative radiograph that confirmed the correct position of the fibula flap

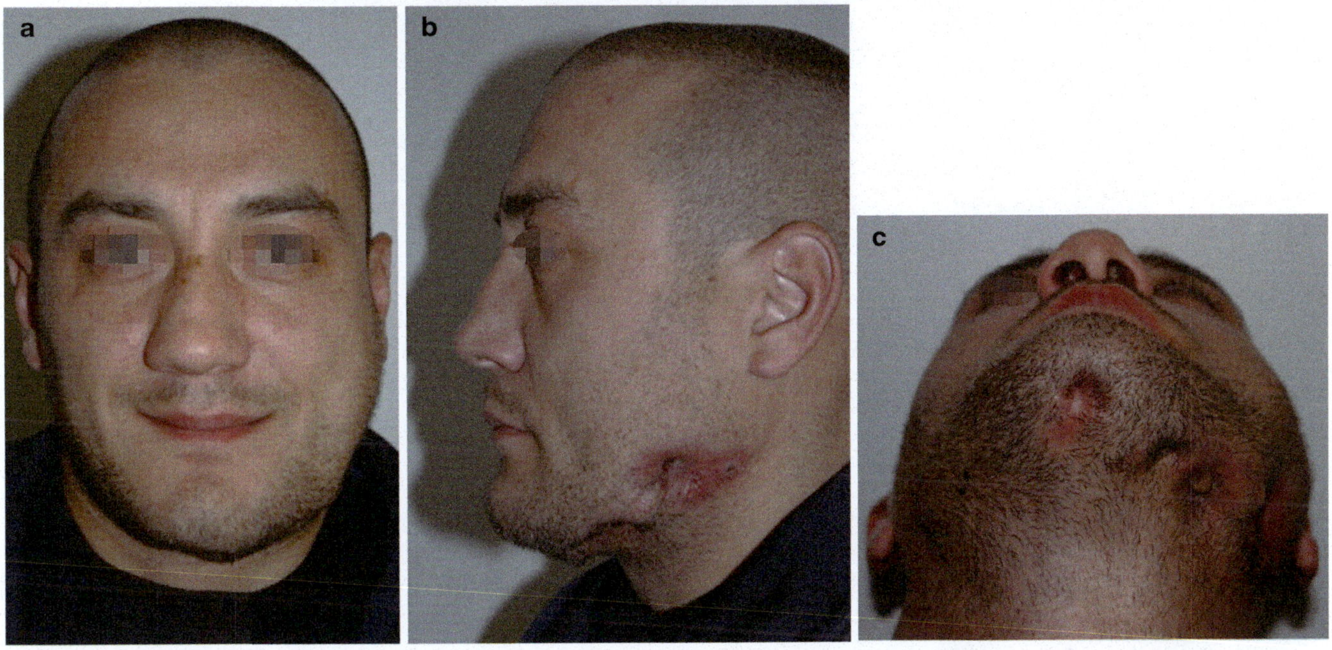

Fig. 7 (**a** and **b**) Frontal and lateral view of patient affected by mandibular chronic osteomyelitis. (**c**) Necrotic bone exposition with surrounding inflammation of the skin and fistulae

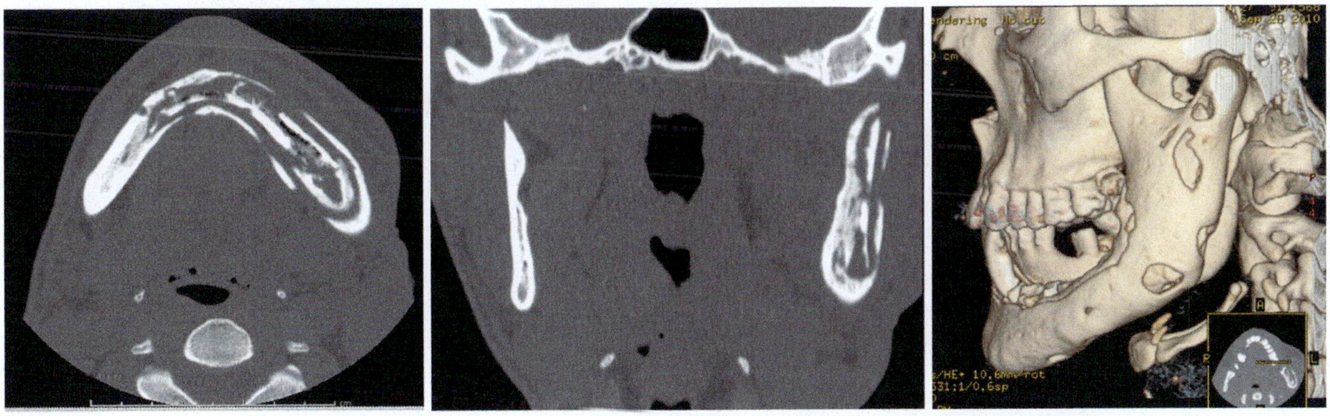

Fig. 8 Axial, coronal view and 3D CT reconstruction. Extensive periosteal reaction extending from the midline of the mandible to the left condyle is evident in keeping with chronic osteomyelitis

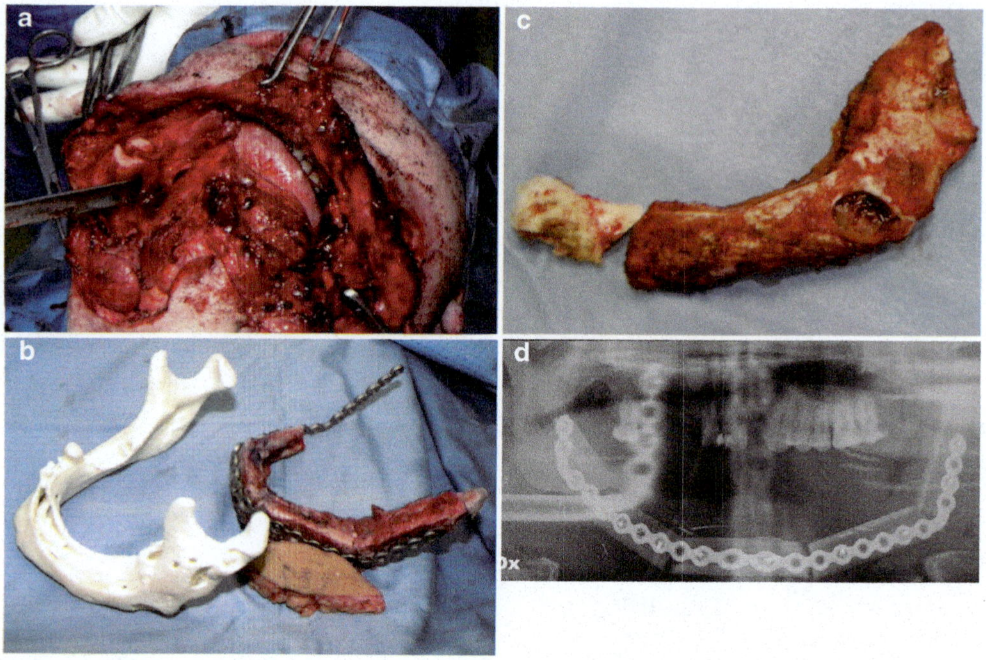

Fig. 9 (**a**) Intraoperative mandibular defect following osteomyelitic bone resection. (**b**) Intraoperative view of malacic bone. (**c**) Intraoperative view of the acrylonitrile butadiene styrene biomodels of the mandible (stereolithography) and the fibula free flap contoured to recreate mandibular shape. (**d**) Postoperative panoramic radiograph depicts the typical configuration of a mandibular arch. The flap is well aligned and held stable by the reconstruction plate

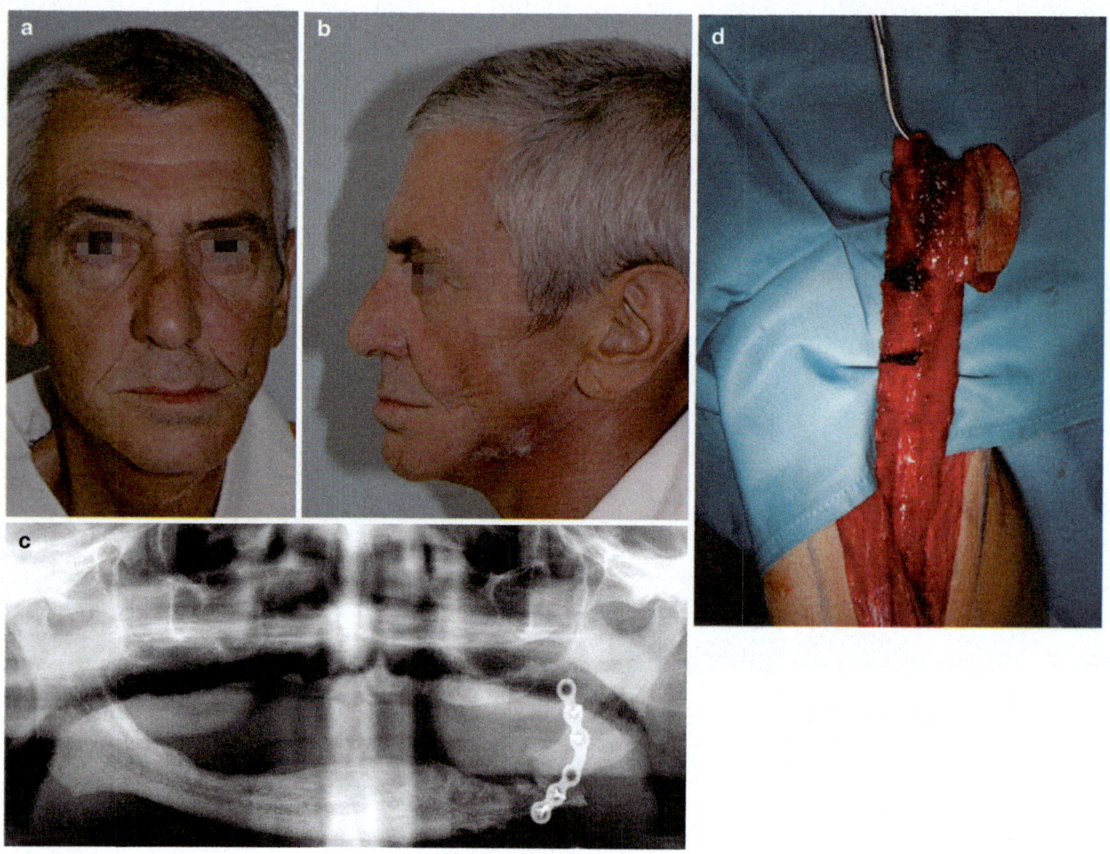

Fig. 10 (**a**) Frontal view of an oncological patient after radiotherapy [20]. (**b**) Lateral view showing bone exposition and fistula through irradiated skin. (**c**) Orthopantomograph showing pathological fracture and plate dislocation of previous mandibulotomy after radiotherapy. (**d**) Osteocutaneous fibula flap was harvested, including the skin paddle. The skin island is located between the middle and distal third of the fibula

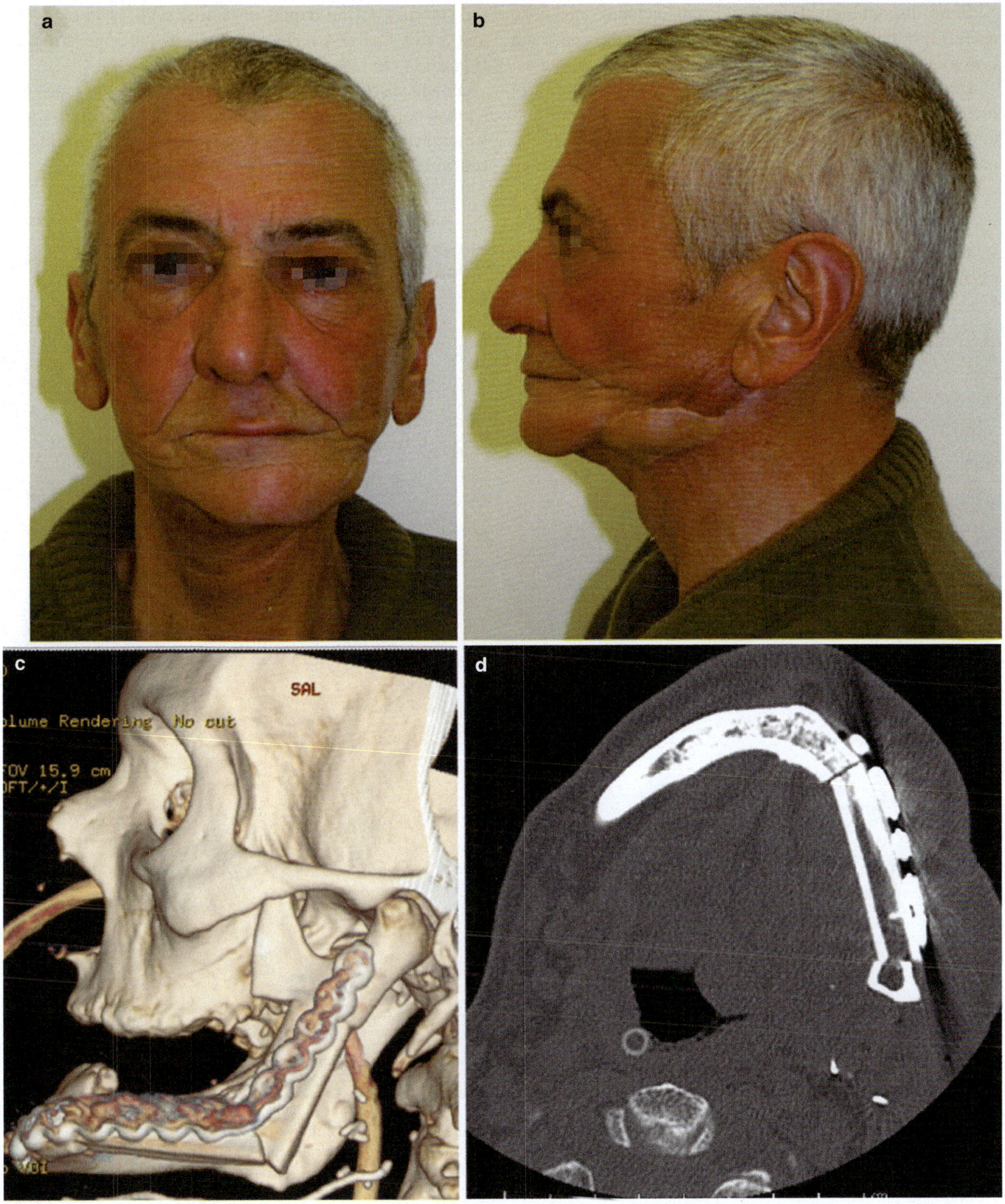

Fig. 11 (**a** and **b**) Frontal and lateral postoperative views. (**c** and **d**) 3D reconstruction and axial view showing mandibular arch reconstruction

Bone discontinuity less than 6 cm includes any bone defects resulting from oncological resection of the upper and lower jaw or congenital malformations such as cleft palate.

Dentoalveolar defects without bone discontinuity include all those cases where, although there are no discontinuities, a bone augmentation is required because the native bone does not have sufficient height to guarantee the stability of the dental implants, such as in classes V and VI of Cawood's classification of jawbone atrophies (Figs. 12–15) [29–31].

Fibula vascularized flaps withstand irradiation much better than bone grafts or plates and, when reconstructing within a previously irradiated field, has the benefit of importing tissue with a new blood supply [32].

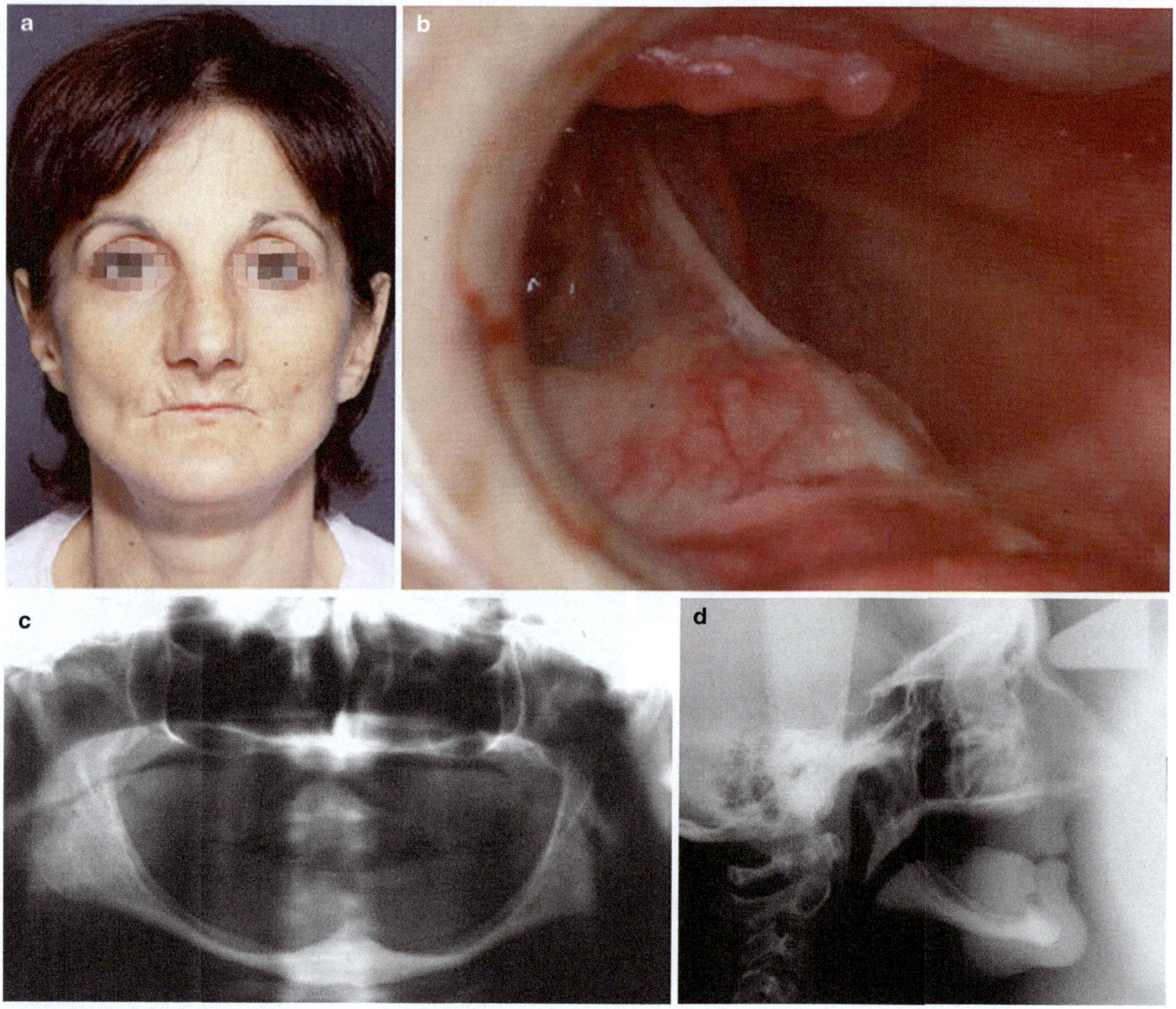

Fig. 12 (**a**) Frontal view of a 48-year-old diabetic and hypothyroid woman with extreme bimaxillary atrophy. (**b**) Intraoral photo showing a severe resorption of both superior and inferior alveolar ridges with complete obliteration of the vestibular fornices. (**c**) Preoperative orthopantomograph. (**d**) Lateral cephalogram showing severe mandibular pseudo-prognathism

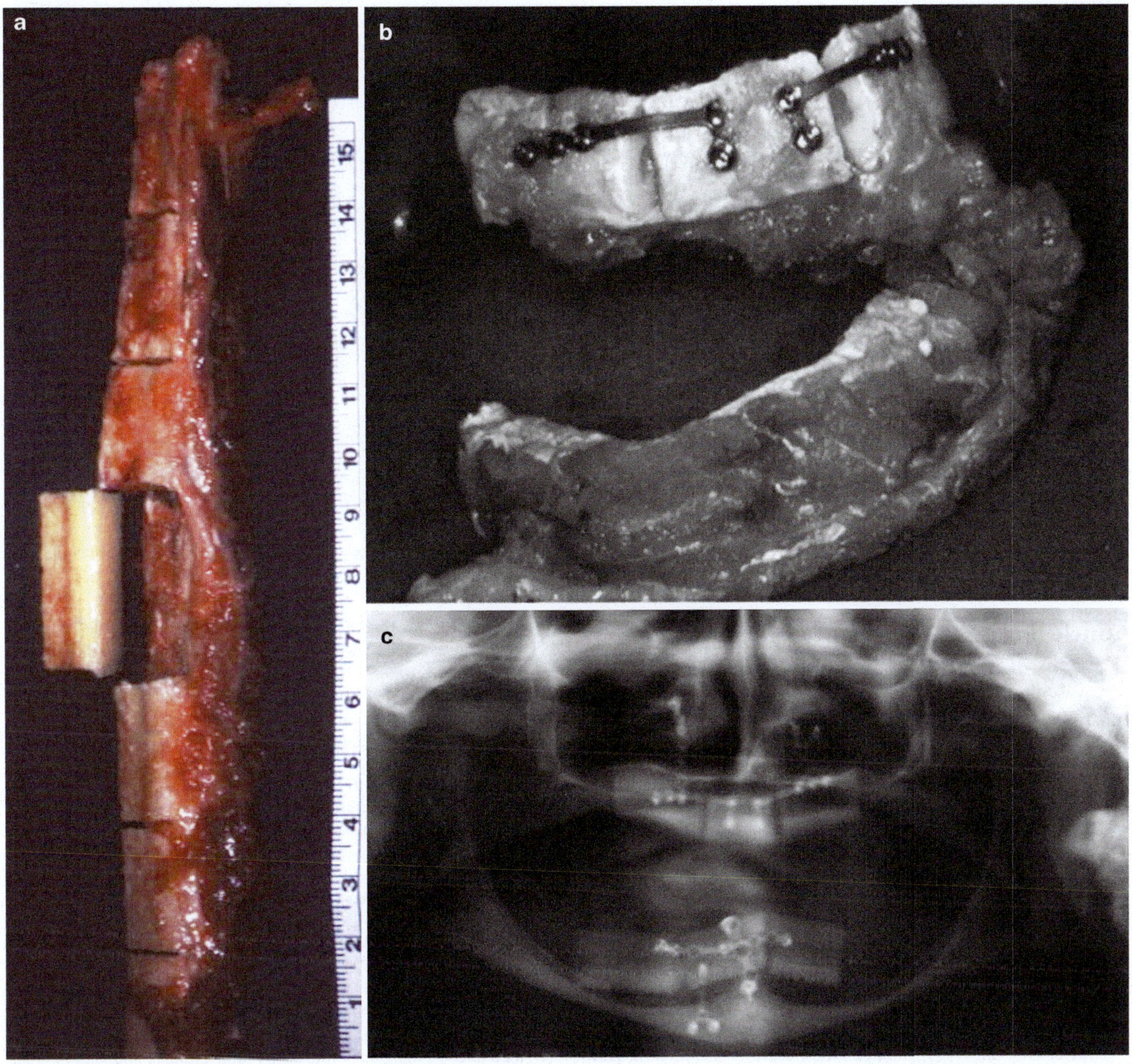

Fig. 13 (**a**) Fibula flap with six osteotomies preserving the periosteal and vascular continuity; a bone segment was removed from the medial third of the fibula leaving the periosteal layer intact. (**b**) Contoured layered fibula flap; three segments were fixed to each other with microplates. (**c**) Postoperative orthopantomograph: the three proximal bone segments, fixed to the mandible, and the three distal segments to the maxilla with microplates

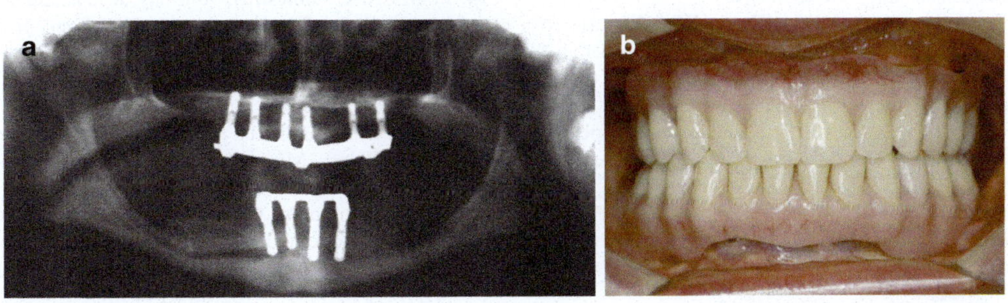

Fig. 14 (**a**) Panoramic radiograph (panorex) demonstrates preservation and union of bone segments with implants in place in reconstructed maxillary and mandibular bones. Notably, the microplates have been removed to facilitate dental implant and prosthetic placement. (**b**) Intraoral view of the implant-supported removable prosthesis [28]

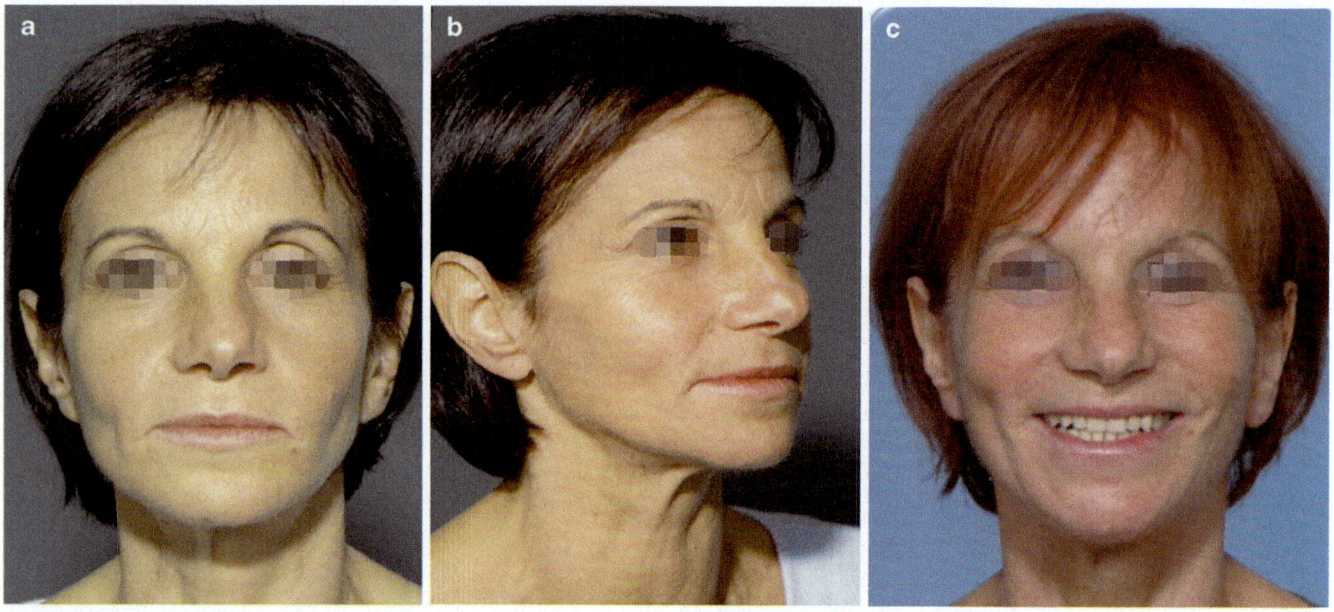

Fig. 15 (**a** and **b**) Four-year posttreatment frontal and lateral view of the patient after reconstruction. (**c**) Ten-year posttreatment frontal view

Conclusion

The vascularized fibula flap has become a flap of choice for most facial reconstructions for several reasons: (1) the ease of harvesting; (2) the availability of lenght and bone quality; (3) the feasibility of obtaining a skin paddle, muscle, or both; (4) the need possibility to perform multiple osteotomies for contouring; (5) the ability to double barrel the flap; (6) the presence of good caliber vessels, including two veins; (7) the probability chance of reliable implant-supported dental rehabilitation; and (8) the presence of minimal donor site morbidity.

References

1. Taylor GI, Miller GD, Ham FJ. The free vascularized bone graft. A clinical extension of microvascular techniques. Plast Reconstr Surg. 1975;55(5):533–44.
2. Chen ZW, Yan W. The study and clinical application of the osteocutaneous flap of fibula. Microsurgery. 1983;4(1):11–6.
3. Hidalgo DA. Fibula free flap: a new method of mandible reconstruction. Plast Reconstr Surg. 1989;84(1):71–9.
4. Cheng MH, Saint-Cyr M, Ali RS, Chang KP, Hao SP, Wei FC. Osteomyocutaneous peroneal artery-based combined flap for reconstruction of composite and en bloc mandibular defects. Head Neck. 2009;31(3):361–70.
5. Heitmann C, Khan FN, Levin LS. Vasculature of the peroneal artery: an anatomic study focused on the perforator vessels. J Reconstr Microsurg. 2003;19(3):157–62.
6. Potter JK, Lee MR, Oxford L, Wong C, Saint-Cyr M. Proximal peroneal perforator in dual-skin paddle configuration of fibula free flap for composite oral reconstruction. Plast Reconstr Surg. 2014;133(6):1485–92.
7. Hayden RE, Mullin DP, Patel AK. Reconstruction of the segmental mandibular defect: current state of the art. Curr Opin Otolaryngol Head Neck Surg. 2012;20(4):231–6.
8. Nocini PF, Saia G, Bettini G, Ragazzo M, Blandamura S, Chiarini L, Bedogni A. Vascularized fibula flap reconstruction of the mandible in bisphosphonate-related osteonecrosis. Eur J Surg Oncol. 2009;35(4):373–9.
9. Chuang DC, Chen HC, Wei FC, Noordhoff MS. Compound functioning free muscle flap transplantation (lateral half of soleus, fibula, and skin flap). Plast Reconstr Surg. 1992;89(2):335–9.
10. Hayden R, O'Leary M. A neurosensory fibula flap: anatomical description and clinical applications. Presented at the 94th annual meeting of the American Laryngological, Rhinological and Otological Society Meeting in Hyatt Regency Waikoloa, Big Island of Hawaii, Hawaii, May 8, 1991.
11. Jones NF, Swartz WM, Mears DC, Jupiter JB, Grossman A. The "double barrel" free vascularized fibular bone graft. Plast Reconstr Surg. 1988;81(3):378–85.
12. Wei FC, Chen HC, Chuang CC, Noordhoff MS. Fibular osteoseptocutaneous flap: anatomic study and clinical application. Plast Reconstr Surg. 1986;78(2):191–200.
13. Foster RD, Anthony JP, Sharma A, Pogrel MA. Vascularized bone flaps versus nonvascularized bone grafts for mandibular reconstruction: an outcome analysis of primary bony union and endosseous implant success. Head Neck. 1999;21(1):66–71.
14. Pogrel MA, Podlesh S, Anthony JP, Alexander J. A comparison of vascularized and nonvascularized bone grafts for reconstruction of mandibular continuity defects. J Oral Maxillofac Surg. 1997;55(11):1200–6.
15. Anesi A, Albanese M, Gerosa R, Corrocher G, Gambarini G, Nocini PF. Mandibular ameloblastic fibroma in 6-years-old girl: a case report. Minerva Stomatol. 2008;57(10):549–55. English, Italian.
16. Anesi A, Bissolotti G, Toller N, Corrocher G, Chiarini L, Nocini PF. O.322 Ameloblastic fibroma in a 6-year-old child: case report. J Craniomaxillofac Surg. 2008;36(Suppl 1):S81. https://doi.org/10.1016/S1010-5182(08)71446-X.

17. Cordeiro PG, Santamaria E. A classification system and algorithm for reconstruction of maxillectomy and midfacial defects. Plast Reconstr Surg. 2000;105(7):2331–46. discussion 2347–8.
18. Cordeiro PG, Chen CM. A 15-year review of midface reconstruction after total and subtotal maxillectomy: part I. Algorithm and outcomes. Plast Reconstr Surg. 2012;129(1):124–36.
19. De Santis G, Nocini PF, Chairini L, Bedogni A. Functional rehabilitation of the atrophic mandible and maxilla with fibula flaps and implant-supported prosthesis. Plast Reconstr Surg. 2004;113(1):88–98. discussion 99–100.
20. Marella GL, Raschellà F, Solinas M, Mutolo P, Potenza S, Milano F, Mauriello S, Caggiano B, Rondinelli P, Anesi A, Migaldi M. The diagnostic delay of oral carcinoma. Ig Sanita Pubbl. 2018;74(3):249–63.
21. Pozzi S, Anesi A, Generali L, Bari A, Consolo U, Chiarini L. Bisphosphonate-related osteonecrosis of the jaw (BRONJ). In: Tsesis I, editor. Complications in endodontic surgery: prevention, identification and management. edn 1 ed. Berlin/Heidelberg: Springer-Verlag; 2014. p. 153–65.
22. Wax MK, Winslow CP, Hansen J, MacKenzie D, Cohen J, Andersen P, Albert T. A retrospective analysis of temporomandibular joint reconstruction with free fibula microvascular flap. Laryngoscope. 2000;110(6):977–81.
23. Chiarini L, Albanese M, Anesi A, Galzignato PF, Mortellaro C, Nocini P, et al. Surgical treatment of unilateral condylar hyperplasia with piezosurgery. J Craniofac Surg. 2014;25:808–10.
24. Chang YM, Wallace CG, Hsu YM, Shen YF, Tsai CY, Wei FC. Outcome of osseointegrated dental implants in double-barrel and vertically distracted fibula osteoseptocutaneous free flaps for segmental mandibular defect reconstruction. Plast Reconstr Surg. 2014;134:1033–43.
25. Nocini PF, Turra M, Valsecchi S, Blandamura S, Bedogni A. Microvascular free bone flap harvest with piezosurgery. J Oral Maxillofac Surg. 2011;69(5):1485–92.
26. Anesi A, Ferretti M, Cavani F, Salvatori R, Bianchi M, Russo A, et al. Structural and ultrastructural analyses of bone regeneration in rabbit cranial osteotomy: Piezosurgery versus traditional osteotomes. J Craniomaxillofac Surg. 2018;46(1):107–18.
27. Turra M, Bertossi D, Bissolotti G, Anesi A, Chiarini L, Nocini PF. O.095 Genioplasty with piezosurgery. J Craniomaxillofac Surg. 2008;36:S24. https://doi.org/10.1016/S1010-5182(08)71219-8.
28. Bertossi D, Bissolotti G, Corrocher G, Anesi A, Nocini PF. O.301 The use of tapered dental implants in severe jaw atrophies. J Craniomaxillofac Surg. 2008;36(Suppl 1):S76. https://doi.org/10.1016/S1010-5182(08)71425-2.
29. Nocini PF, De Santis G, Bedogni A, Chiarini L. Simultaneous bimaxillary alveolar ridge augmentation by a single free fibular transfer: a case report. J Craniomaxillofac Surg. 2002;30:46–53.
30. Cawood JI, Howell RA. A classification of the edentulous jaws. Int J Oral Maxillofac Surg. 1988;17(4):232–6.
31. Rohner D, Bucher P, Kunz C, Hammer B, Schenk RK, Prein J. Treatment of severe atrophy of the maxilla with the prefabricated free vascularized fibula flap. Clin Oral Implants Res. 2002;13(1):44–52.
32. Kim JW, Hwang JH, Ahn KM. Fibular flap for mandible reconstruction in osteoradionecrosis of the jaw: selection criteria of fibula flap. Maxillofac Plast Reconstr Surg. 2016;38(1):46.

Evolution in Preoperative Imaging

Massimo Pinelli, Alberto Puglisi, and Giorgio De Santis

The microvascular free fibula flap is currently one of the preferred methods for reconstruction of the oromandibular defect. The patency of the major vessels in the donor lower limb should be evaluated before the fibula is harvested because the blood supply can be inadequate for safe utilization of this flap.

History and physical examination are not helpful in detecting most congenital vascular and bone anomalies that would place the foot at high risk for ischemia if the peroneal artery is sacrificed.

The extent of preoperative technological assessment prior to performing a fibula free flap is controversial. Some authors do not think that routine pre-op imaging is indicated [1, 2]. They reserve angiography for evaluation of patients with abnormal distal pulses or history of lower limbs trauma. Imaging does, however, detect congenital and acquired abnormalities in lower extremities (bone, vessels, muscles, etc.; Figs. 1 and 2) that may be overlooked on clinical evaluation. Patients undergoing a partial jawbone reconstruction are often at high risk for peripheral vascular disease due to smoking and advanced age. Significant atherosclerotic disease may be detected, and this suggests the side of fibula harvest or the need for alternative reconstructions. Bone and vascular disorders could greatly affect the final result and could expose the patient to very important complications. This is the reason that instrumental investigations are so important before surgery. Both the recipient and the donor area must be studied. Normally, the oromandibular region is thoroughly investigated to delineate the area of the disease and to determine the size of the defect (Fig. 3); the leg from which the fibula free flap is harvested must also be exhaustively investigated to assess if the area is eligible and will not cause complication to the foot. The first evaluation is a bone investigation (see Fig. 2) to verify if bone alterations are present due to congenital disease or post-traumatic outcome. The key point of the investigation remains the vascular supply to the foot.

If congenital variations of the popliteal artery branches are detected in femoral angiograms (diagnosed in 7.8% of

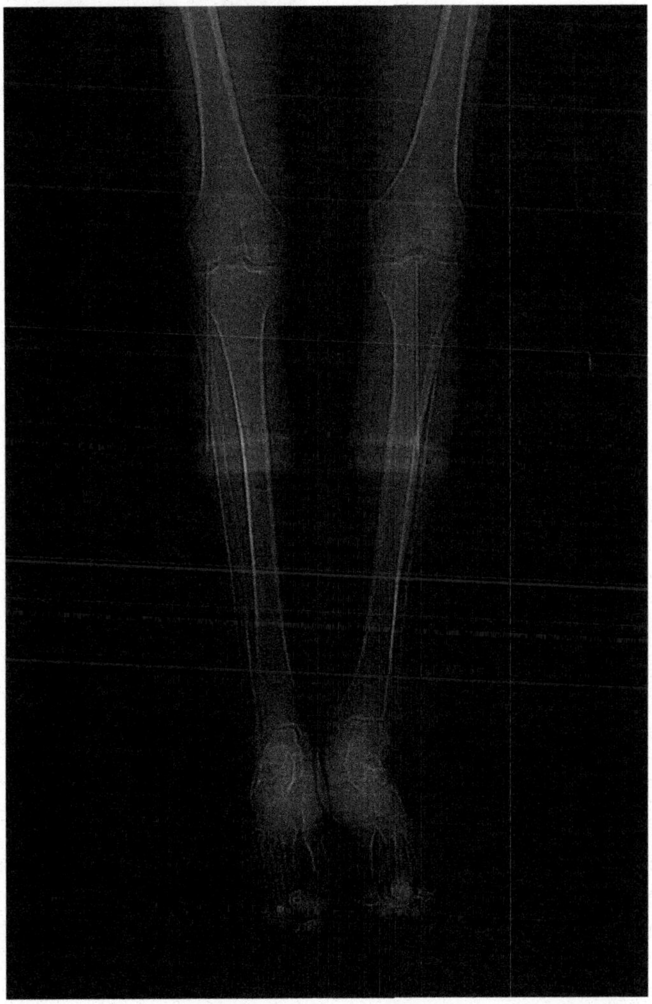

Fig. 1 CT scan of the fibula

M. Pinelli · A. Puglisi · G. De Santis (✉)
Plastic and Reconstructive Surgery Unit, University Hospital of Modena, Modena, Italy
e-mail: pinelli.massimo@aou.mo.it; desantis.giorgio@unimore.it

G. De Santis et al. (eds.), *Atlas of Mandibular and Maxillary Reconstruction with the Fibula Flap*,
https://doi.org/10.1007/978-3-030-10684-3_9

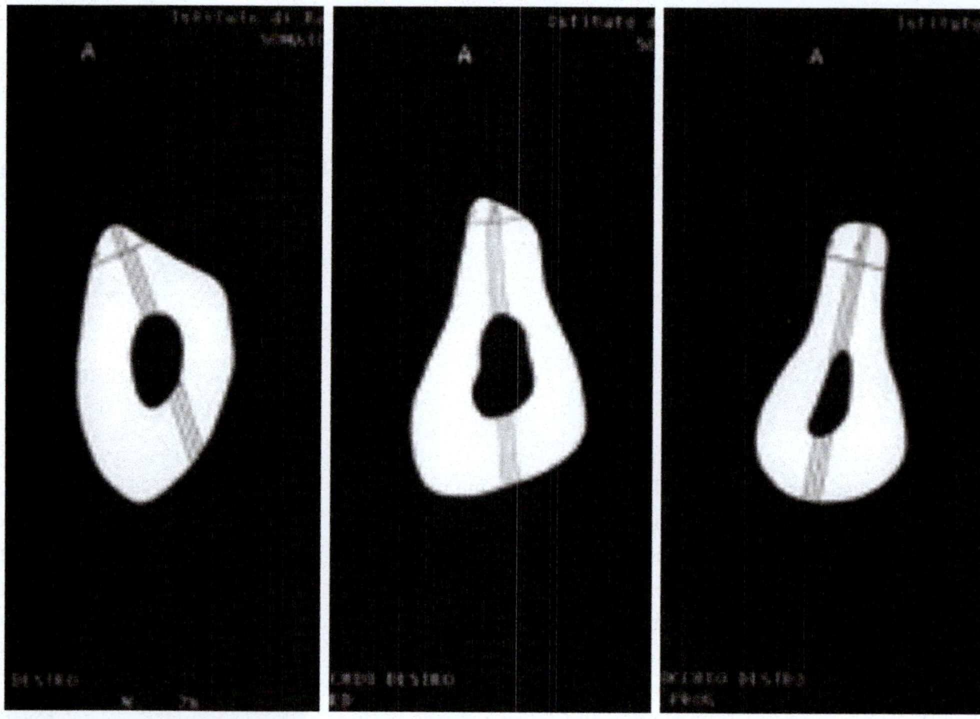

Fig. 2 CT scan of the fibula at increasingly distal levels

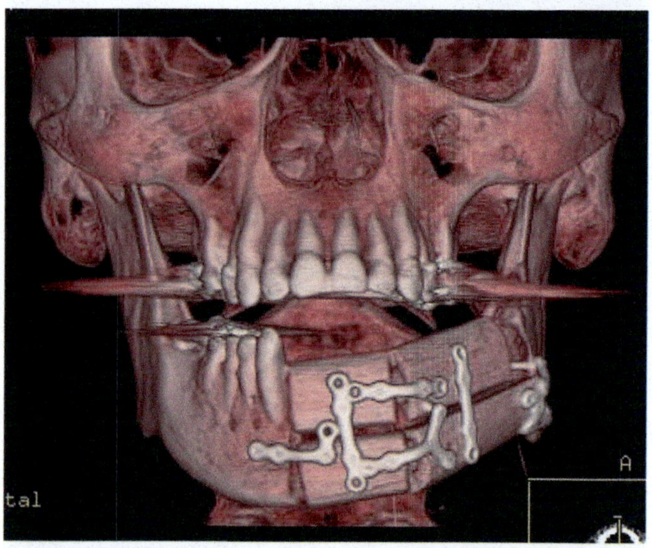

Fig. 3 3D CT scan of double-barrel reconstruction for full height mandibular defects

patients) [3], the reconstructive plan may need to be revised. Congenital absence of peroneal artery is rare (incidence 0.1%) [4]. Serious complications may also result if the peroneal artery is the dominant vascular supply to the foot, which has been reported in 5–7% of the population [3, 5, 6].

Candidates with peroneal artery magna are at high risk for ischemia with fibula free flaps. This congenital anomaly occurs in 0.2–0.9% of the population. These patients have normal pulses and are without claudication despite having the peroneal artery as the sole arterial supply of the foot [2, 3, 7, 8].

Overall, imaging has been reported to change the reconstructive plan of 21–25% of patients being evaluated for fibula free flap [8, 9].

The best method for preoperative evaluation of the lower limb vasculature is controversial. Femoral angiography has been considered as the gold standard; the current literature, however, advocates less invasive methods of assessment such as magnetic resonance angiography and color flow Doppler.

With its high positive predictive value and sensitivity, preoperative CT-angiography can improve the chances of a successful outcome. It provides the reconstructive surgeon with a road map, revealing vasculature anomalies or disease that could alter or contraindicate surgery.

Angiography is considered the procedure of choice by many surgeons for evaluating the anatomy of arteries [8–10]. Digital subtraction angiography provides accurate, detailed, functional anatomy of lower extremity vessels. Disadvantages include expense and the risk of complications such as hemorrhage, thrombosis, embolism, pseudoaneurysm, arteriovenous fistula, and allergic reactions [11].

Magnetic resonance angiography is a noninvasive alternative for preoperative vasculature examination. This investigation has a cost similar to that of conventional angiography and is capable of identifying vasculature anomalies [12].

Color flow Doppler studies have been proposed as an inexpensive and accurate method of evaluating lower extremity vasculature. Color flow Doppler has a sensitivity for detecting 95% of occluded vessels and 87% of stenotic vessels [13]. According to some authors, patients with monophasic flow or no flow in any of the trifurcation vessels have a high risk of ischemic complications. Patients with biphasic flow require evaluation with CT angiography, MR angiography, or angiography, and patients with triphasic flow do not require any further evaluation [14].

Current common practice is MR angiography for patients undergoing jaw reconstruction using fibula free flap. This investigation provides the most detailed information about the anatomy of lower extremity vasculature.

It is considered safe to harvest a fibula free flap in patients with two-vessel runoff, provided that the patent's tibial vessel is the dominant arterial supply to the foot. In addition, there must be a well-defined vessel at the level of the ankle (distal to the proposed peroneal artery harvest) from the remaining tibial vessel to the obstructed tibio-peroneal territory. Other reconstructive options must be considered in patients whose peroneal artery is the dominant or sole artery to the foot.

Despite the precautions described herein, a small risk of donor site morbidity, including foot loss, remains. This is true of any fibula flap transfer. CT angiography may be used as a screen depending on surgeon preference. If three-vessel runoff is detected, then no further investigations are required. If two-vessel runoff is noted, an angiogram is strongly recommended to establish with as much certainty as possible whether flap harvest will be safe.

In conclusion, a fibula free flap can be safely performed in patients with three-vessel runoff or in patients with two-vessel runoff provided that the tibial artery is the dominant arterial supply to the foot.

Angiography provides accurate detail of the arterial supply to the lower limbs.

Computer-aided design (CAD) and computer-aided manufacturing (CAM) have recently opened new frontiers for surgeons. CAD/CAM procedure guides the surgeon in correctly positioning the residual bone and fibula free flap in secondary mandibular reconstruction. In this procedure, high-resolution CT is the key point to getting a virtual surgical plan. A virtual surgical guide is projected to aid the repositioning of the bone segments in their original locations, and a computer reconstruction bone plate is provided to support the fibula free flap (CAD). The stereolithographic files of the guide and plate are then printed three-dimensionally (CAM) [15] (Figs. 4 and 5).

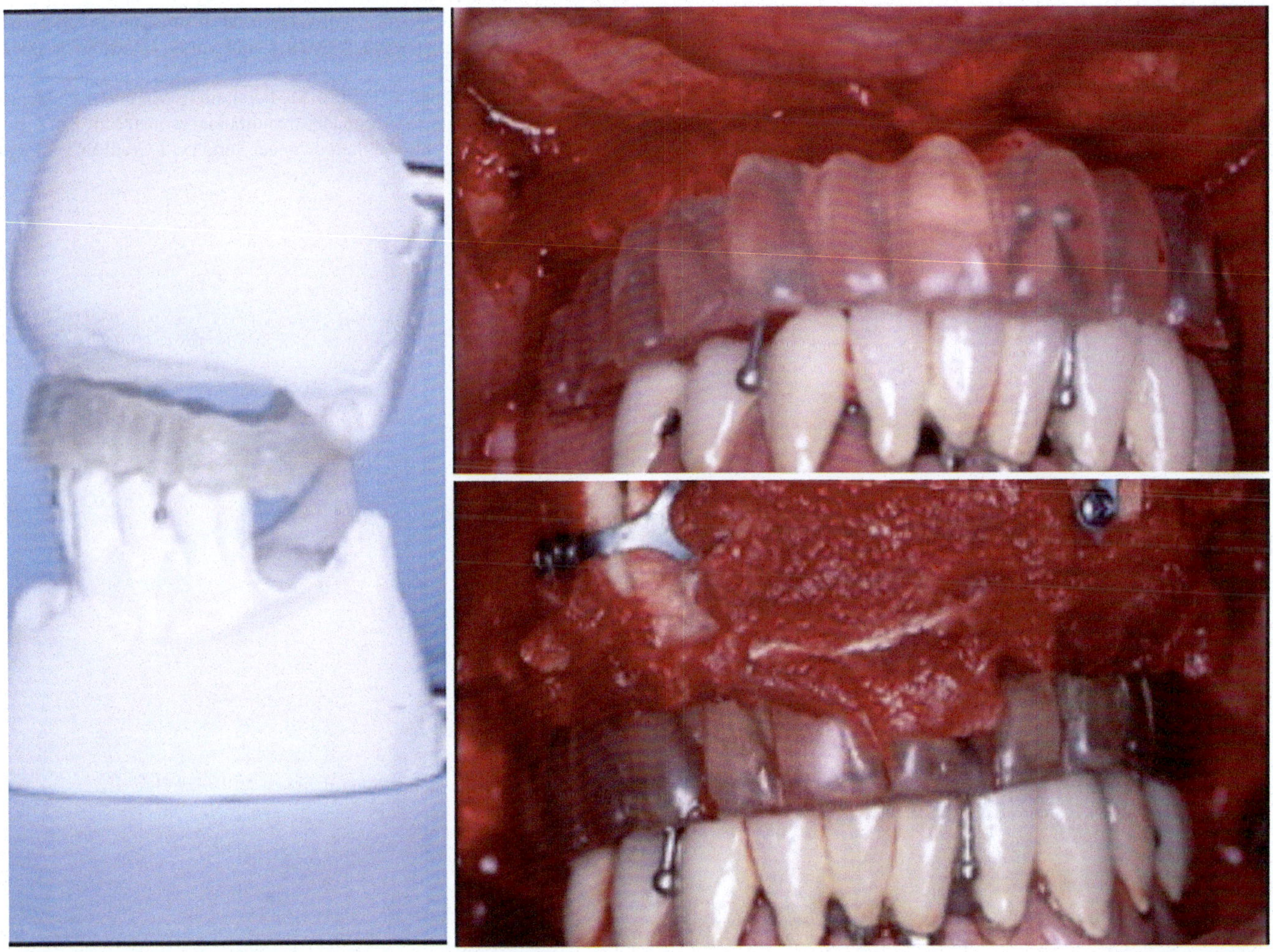

Fig. 4 Splint fabrication for the benefit of accurate intraoperative flap insetting (case of maxilla reconstruction)

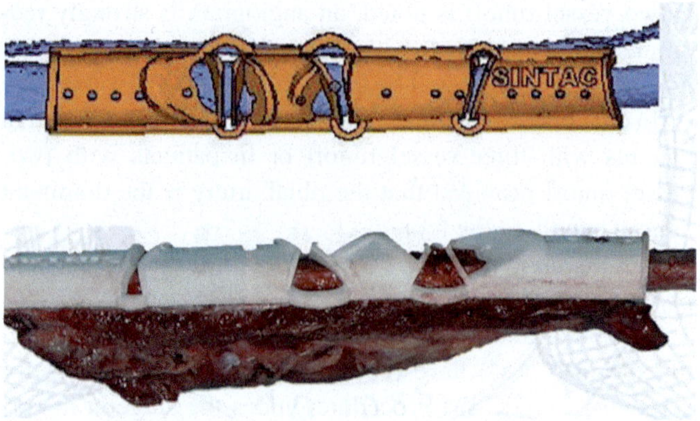

Fig. 5 Surgical cutting guide for the fibula, determining the exact location and indication of osteotomies when applied on the donor bone

This recent technology allows the appropriate bone-plate relationship, a good functional outcome, and a correct occlusion (see Fig. 3).

References

1. Yim KK, Wei FC. Fibula osteoseptocutaneous flap for mandible reconstruction. Microsurgery. 1994;15:245–9.
2. Disa JJ, Cordeiro PG. The current role of preoperative arteriography in fibula free flaps. Plast Reconstr Surg. 1998;102:1083–8.
3. Kim D, Orron DE, Skillman JJ. Surgical significance of popliteal artery variants: a unified angiographic classification. Ann Surg. 1989;210:776–81.
4. Lippert H, Pabst R. Arterial variations in man: classification and frequency. New York: JF Bergman Verlag; 1985. p. 60–3.
5. Kadir S. Arterial anatomy of the trunk and extremities. In: Kadir S, Brothers MF, editors. Atlas of normal and variant angiographic anatomy. Philadelphia: WB Saunders Co; 1991. p. 124.
6. Yamada T, Gloviczi P, Bower TC, Naessens JM, Carmichael SW. Variations of arterial anatomy of the foot. Am J Surg. 1993;166:130–5.
7. Lutz BS, Wei FC, Ng SH, Chen SHT. Routine donor leg angiography before vascularized free fibula transfer is not necessary: a prospective study in 120 clinical cases. Plast Reconstr Surg. 1999;103:121–7.
8. Young DM, Trabulsy PP, Anthony JP. The need for preoperative leg angiography in fibula free flaps. J Reconstr Microsurg. 1994;10:283–9.
9. Blackwell KE. Donor site evaluation for fibula free flap transfer. Am J Otolaryngol. 1998;19:89–95.
10. Klein S, Hage JJ, van der Horst CM, Lagerweij M. Ankle-arm index versus angiography for the reassessment of fibula free flap. Last Reconstr Surg. 2003;111:735–43.
11. Hessel SJ, Adams DF, Abrams HL. Complications of angiography. Radiology. 1981;138:273–81.
12. Manaste BJ, Coleman DA, Bell DA. Magnetic resonance imaging of vascular anatomy before vascularized fibula grafting. J Bone Joint Surg Am. 1990;72:409–14.
13. Polak JF. Peripheral arterial disease: evaluation with color flow and duplex sonography. Radiol Clin N Am. 1995;33:71–90.
14. Smith RB, Thomas RD, Funk GF. Fibula free flaps: the role of angiography in patients with abnormal results on preoperative color flow doppler studies. Arch Otolaryngol Head Neck Surg. 2003;129:712–5.
15. Ciocca L, Mazzoni S, Fantini M, Persiani F, Marchetti C, Scotti R. CAD/CAM guided secondary mandibular reconstruction of a discontinuity defect after ablative cancer surgery. J Craniomaxillofac Surg. 2012;40:e511–5.

Evolution in Bone Synthesis

Andrea Fior, Alexandre Anesi, and Pier Francesco Nocini

Wound coverage, restoring the continuity of jaws, supporting the airway, restoring facial contour, and providing a biologic base for dental rehabilitation are objectives of reconstruction in both mandible and maxilla [1].

Most authors agree that vascularized bone is need for optimal reconstruction of jaw defect, while the debate is still open on the fixation method with free fibula flap [2].

The difficulty with the fixation method in jaws reconstruction with fibula flap is related to the number of osteotomies required and the length of the bone segments needed. The larger the defect in the jaw, the more osteotomies are necessary, and the more complex the procedure becomes. Length and angle of the bone segments have a direct effect on their position, which affect the final facial bone contour (i.e., chin, upper lip, zygoma, orbital rim).

Generally speaking, fixation techniques can be divided into rigid and nonrigid forms of fixation.

Nonrigid Fixation

Nonrigid fixation uses interosseous wire fixation, wire mesh fixation, overlay and onlay bone grafting, titanium tray fixation, and Kirschner wire fixation. Interosseous wires can sometimes be augmented by Kirschner wire fixation (Figs. 1–7) [3]. Intermaxillary fixation after surgery (held for 2 weeks) often provides additional stability when a nonrigid fixation method is used [4]. In the late 1980s and 1990s, interosseous wires were the most common method of fixation. If more than one osteotomy is necessary, the shaping of fibula segments and fixation by wires can be a laborious and difficult procedure. Accurate contact between the bone segments is a major determinant of success of the wiring technique. It is difficult, however, to stabilize a multiple osteotomized graft with wires, especially in the case of mandible reconstruction [4]. Studies have not been able to demonstrate any difference in the rate of bone healing between the rigid and nonrigid fixation methods (94% vs 96%) in mandibular reconstruction, but interosseous wire fixation shows relatively fewer complications (infections and soft tissue damage). The authors conclude, however, by recommending reconstruction plates because they are less laborious than wire fixation [5, 6]. The rich blood supply of a vascularized bone graft is likely the reason for this good outcome with wires, which is significantly different from a fractured atrophic edentulous mandible treated by nonrigid fixation [7]. Nevertheless, nonrigid fixation methods are rarely used in today's clinical practice, because they prove to be laborious.

Rigid Fixation

Rigid fixation methods use lag screw fixation, staples, titanium tray fixation, external fixation appliances, miniplates, and diverse reconstruction plates.

Capizzi et al. described the use of lag screws for fixation at the junctions between the remaining mandible and the transferred fibula flap bone [8]. A lag screw inserted at right angles to the fracture plane provides maximum interfragmental compression but minimal axial stability. Therefore, ideally, one screw should be at a right angle to the long axis and the other at a right angle to the fracture plane [9]. The lag screw technique affects only the periosteum under the head of the lag screw, optimizing the blood supply to the remainder of the vascularized bone graft. Condylar head, condylar neck, and superior ramus are areas of limited exposure; the lag screw technique is appropriate because reducing the

A. Fior · P. F. Nocini (✉)
Division of Oral and Maxillo-Facial Surgery, University Hospital of Modena, Verona, Italy
e-mail: andrea.fior@aovr.veneto.it; pierfrancesco.nocini@univr.it

A. Anesi
Cranio-Maxillo-Facial Surgery Unit, University Hospital of Modena, Modena, Italy
e-mail: alexandre.anesi@unimore.it

G. De Santis et al. (eds.), *Atlas of Mandibular and Maxillary Reconstruction with the Fibula Flap*, https://doi.org/10.1007/978-3-030-10684-3_10

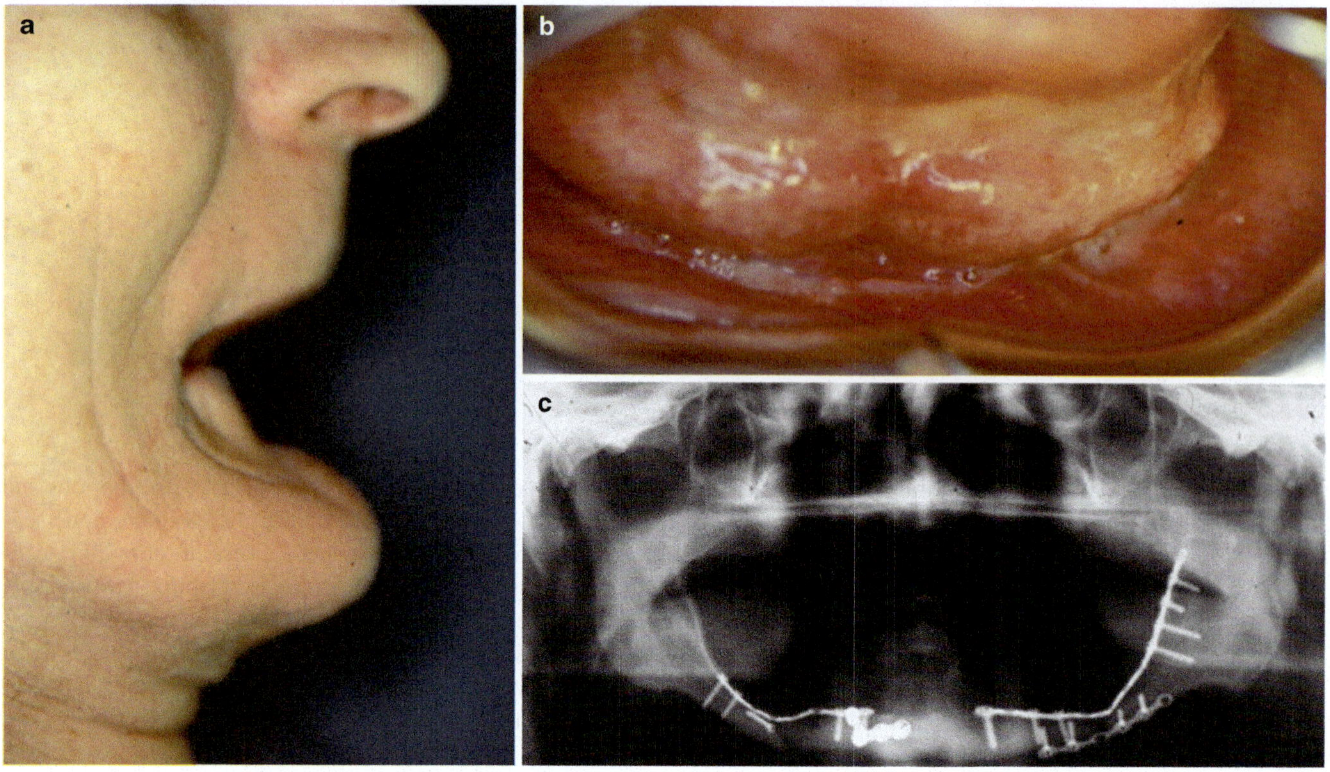

Fig. 1 (**a**) Patient profile. Extreme atrophy of the lower jaw. (**b**) Intraoral view in which the mouth floor is vertically higher respect to basal mandible bone. (**c**) Orthopantomograph of mandible fixed with titanium plates after previous pathological fracture

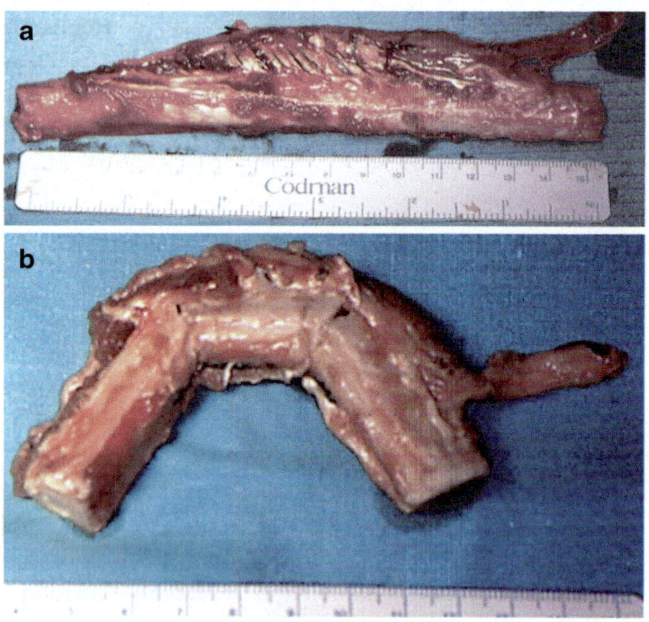

Fig. 2 (**a**) Fibula flap harvested (clinical case dating to 1992). (**b**) Contoured fibula flap for mandible restoration

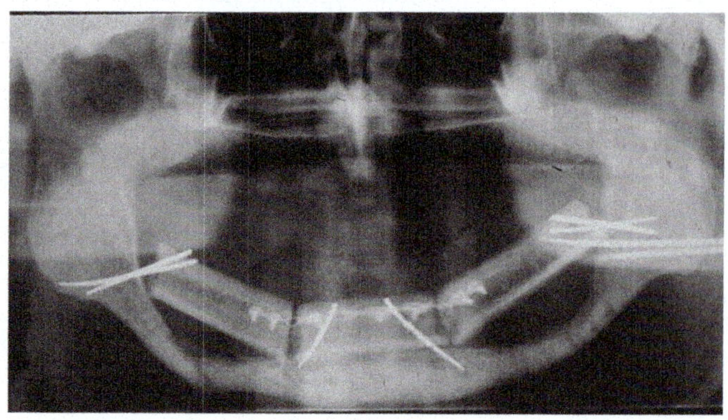

Fig. 3 Postoperative orthopantomograph. Fixation of fibula flap to natural mandible was carried out by Kirschner's wires. Intersegmental fixation was carried out by miniplates

periosteal elevation is required for plate fixation. However, wedge osteotomies for contouring the fibula were done by Capizzi et al. through miniplates (Figs. 8 and 9) [8]. Most surgeons prefer a single fixation method for fibula insetting time, while lag screws need to be associated with miniplates. In today's practice, lag screw fixation for the fibula is not the first choice of most reconstructive teams.

Nickel-titanium (NiTi) alloy staples suitable for use in mandibular fracture have also been described [10]. In mandibular reconstruction with free fibula flap, Strackee and co-authors reported fixation by staples in association with miniplates, not at the junctions of the natural mandible but at the wedge of intersegmental osteotomies. Reported advantages of staple fixation include that it has a minimal effect on the periosteal blood supply and that little dissection is necessary to place drill holes. A particular characteristic of the

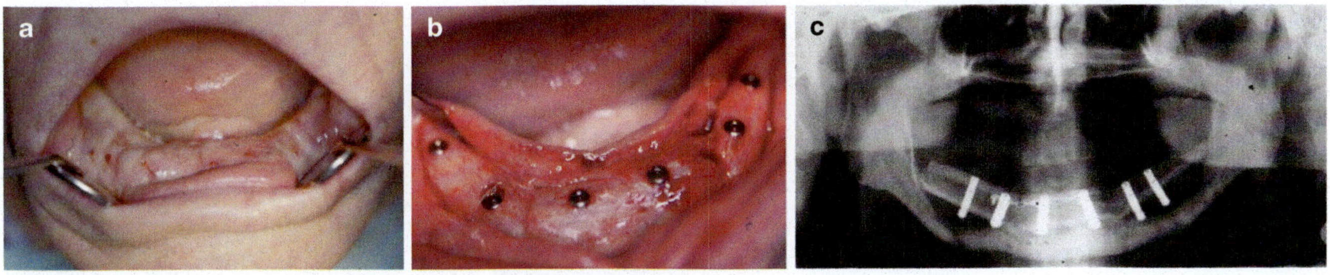

Fig. 4 (**a**) Intraoral view of healed fibula flap. (**b**) Dental endosseous implant were placed in the reconstructed alveolar bone. (**c**) Orthopantomograph after dental implant placement. Note the bicortical placement of dental implants

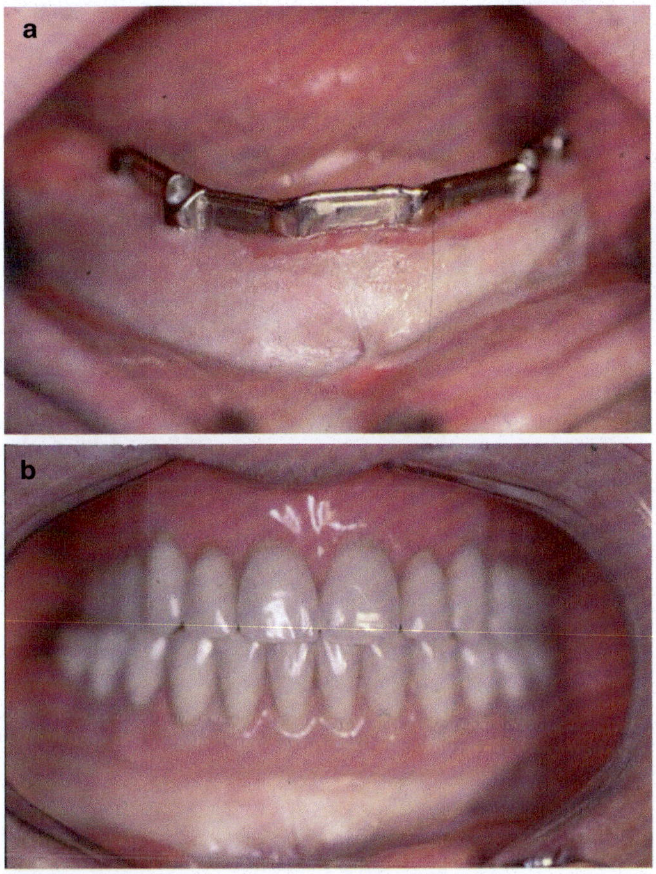

Fig. 5 (**a**) The metalwork is in situ on the top of the abutments. Note the reconstructed inferior vestibular fornix reconstructed with split-thickness skin graft. (**b**) In situ dental implant-borne prosthetic rehabilitation

NiTi alloy is the shape-memory effect: its shape is temperature dependent. The fixation material has less bulk compared to plates, thus reducing the need for its removal in case of dental implants [3]. These fixation devices are not very common in clinical practice, however, because a second fixation method is needed to stabilize the bone graft at locations other than the junctions of the natural mandible. Staples are rarely used in reconstructive surgery of the jaws with fibula flap, as compared to their frequency of use in orthopedics.

Although various techniques have been reported in the literature, the current most common method of establishing bony fixation to the remaining mandible is the use of titanium plates and screws [1, 2, 4, 5, 11, 12].

Following on improvement in hardware technology, several reconstruction plate systems have been described: Arbeitsgemeinschaft für Osteosynthesefragen (AO) stainless steel, AO titanium, and titanium hollow screw reconstruction plate (THORP). These have all been progressively dismissed because of complications. THORP, for example, was abandoned owing to its large screw diameter, plate profile height, and difficulties in hardware removal. The locking screw technology of the THORP system gave rise to the modern locking mandibular reconstruction plate (LMRP), which is one of the most important technological advances in mandibular fixation (Fig. 10). The LMRP offers several theoretical advantages over pre-existing systems, including the need for fewer osteosyntheses and fewer screws [2, 11]. With LMRP it becomes unnecessary for the plate to intimately contact the underlying bone in all areas, thus avoiding compression of periosteal blood perfusion of the underlying cortical bone [13]. Loose screws and non-union are rare complications of LMRP, while the incidence of hardware removal was much higher with respect to miniplates; however, this last problem is related to patients who have a history of radiation therapy and cancer recurrence [2]. Lower-profile locking reconstruction plates and smaller screw diameters were an evolution of LMRP for reducing hardware height that can distort the mandible contour (mostly the chin) [2, 3]. Farwell et al. demonstrated that there was no significant difference in the complication rate between the lower-profile and higher-profile reconstruction plates [14].

Disadvantages of rigid reconstruction plates in fibula fixation include increased cost, procedure complexity, hardware exposure, difficulty in applying large screws to thin cortices, interference with the vascular pedicle, and problems of metal fatigue when bending plates in the sagittal plane [11, 12, 15, 16].

Even with lower-profile locking reconstruction plates, the hardware volume often compromises dental implant positioning for oral rehabilitation. When an opportunity for reopera-

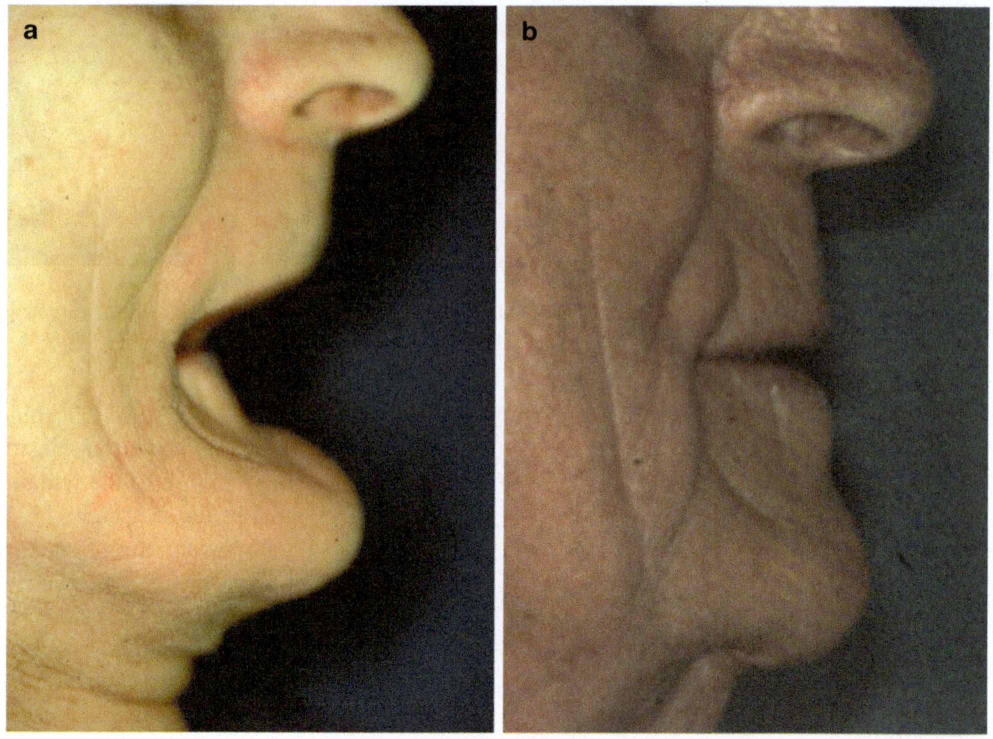

Fig. 6 Preoperative (**b**) and postoperative (**b**) patient profile. A reverse lifting effect was obtained through fibula flap and implant-borne prosthetic rehabilitation

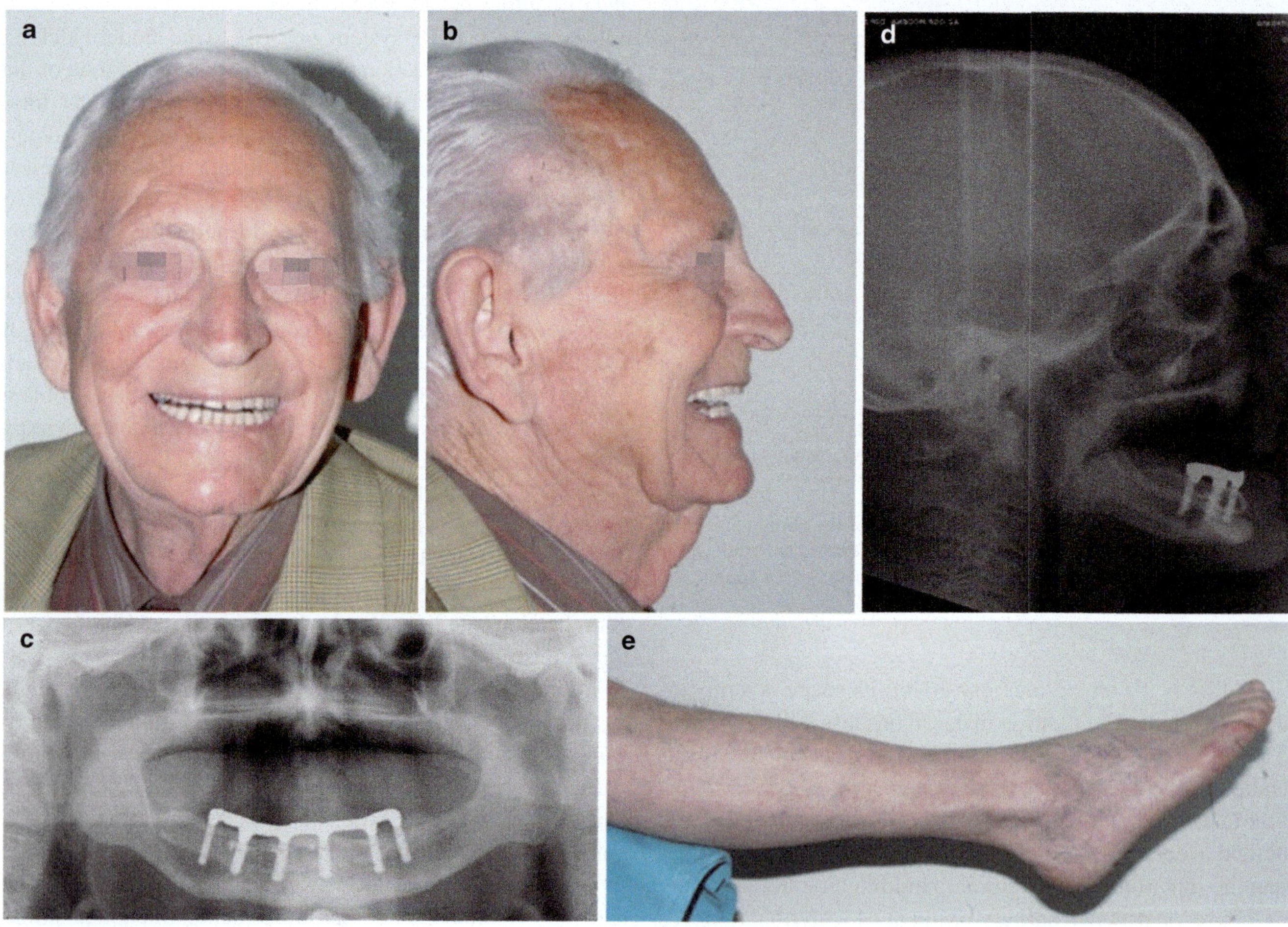

Fig. 7 (**a**, **b**) Final patient aspect after 28 years of masticatory load. (**c**) Current orthopantomograph. The gap between the bone fibula flap and the mandible is filled with spontaneous bone regeneration. (**d**) Final lateral teleradiograph. (**e**) No functional deficits are detectable at the donor leg

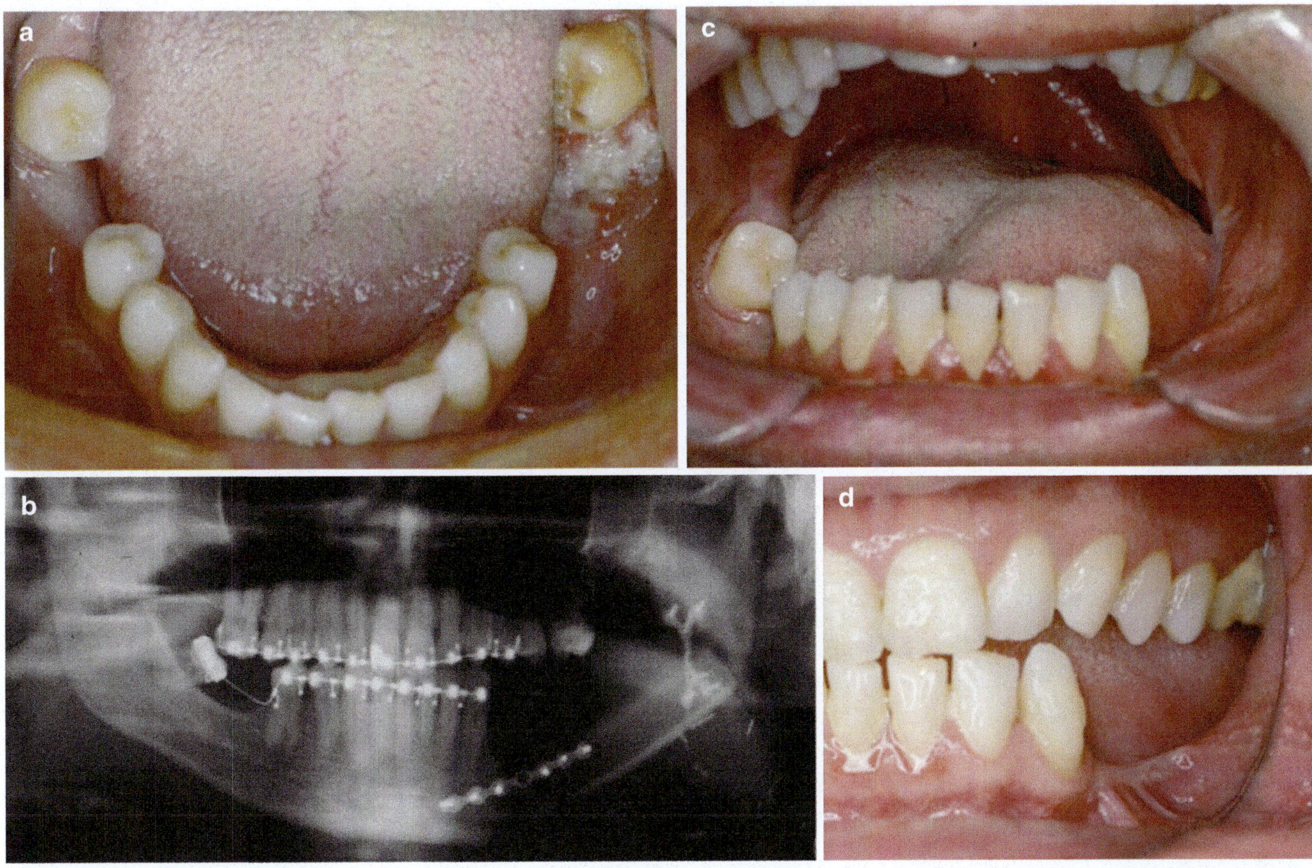

Fig. 8 (**a**) Left retromolar trigone cancer. (**b**) The lateral mandible defect includes the body and angle, which corresponds to a Type IIIB defect (according to P.G. Cordeiro's classification); postoperative orthopantomograph. (**c**) Postoperative intraoral view with effective mouth opening. (**d**) No intraoral skin paddle was used

Fig. 9 Preoperative (**a**) and postoperative (**b**) frontal views of the patient

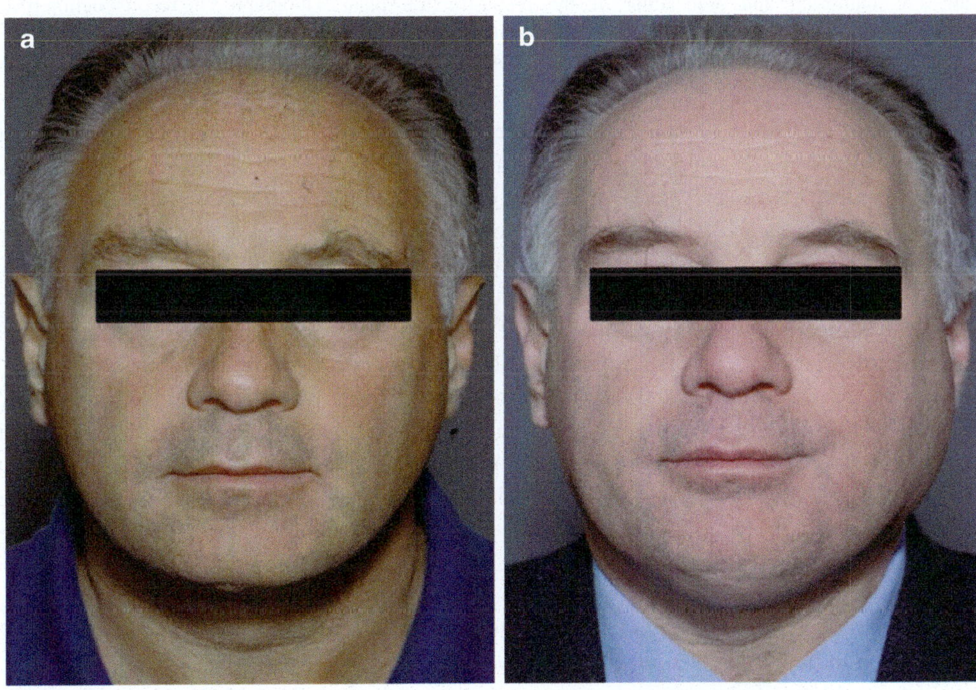

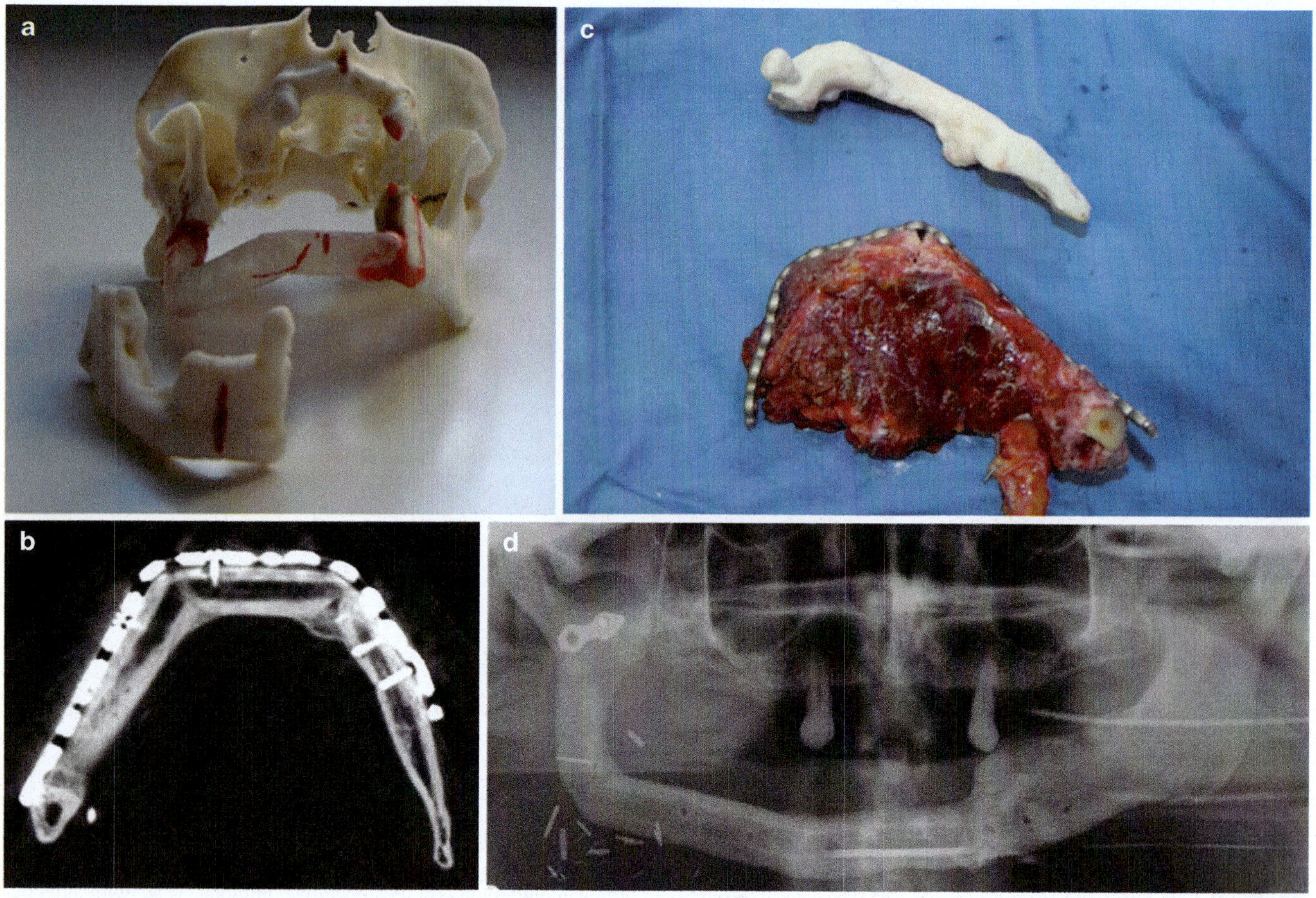

Fig. 10 (**a**) Stereolithographic model of the mandible for preoperative simulation of the resection. We performed a manufacture of an acrylic surgical template for reconstruction that considered the dental model as well. Pre-contouring and prebending of the reconstruction plate (2.7 mm) was carried out according to the acrylic surgical template, outside the operation theater; afterward the fixation hardware was sterilized and was ready for the intervention. (**b**) Bone union occurred uneventfully. (**c**) Comparison between the planned resection and the contoured fibula flap with a reconstruction plate. (**d**) Final orthopantomograph. The reconstruction plate was removed for endosseous dental implant positioning. The prosthodontic plan was suspended because the patient developed cerebral strokes

tion or dental implant positioning arises, plates are removed after bony union. Late complications and complaints about palpable hardware are so prevented by removal of plates. Once the plate has been taken off, the mandibular contour can also improve. Extensive approach and incision are usually needed to remove the reconstruction plate, while smaller incisions are required for select removal of miniplates [1, 11, 12, 15].

Plate exposure was a problem regardless of the particular plate used. However, in mandibular reconstruction with vascularized fibula, conservative wound care after plate exposure often led to healing by secondary intention and to plate coverage, thanks to the high trophism characteristic of composite revascularized flaps [11].

The maintenance of condyle positioning is fundamental in mandible reconstruction. This aim can be achieved by contouring the reconstruction bar over the natural mandible, prior to mandibular resection. Temporary preoperative maxillo-mandibular fixation (steel wire) is often useful, in our experience, for proper positioning of the bone flap with maintenance of condyle position. When possible, this technique works well with reconstruction plates and some longer miniplate systems [3, 11, 15]. In our opinion, intraoperative external fixation systems are cumbersome [17]. Accurate planning for contouring and positioning of the reconstruction plate can simplify the procedure.

The reconstruction plate can usually be contoured prior to mandibular resection, working as a template fixed to the remaining mandibular abutments, within which the fibula flap is given a contour for subsequent fixation with locking screws [3, 11, 15]. This procedure, however, needs surgical time for repeated contouring of bone segments until they are thoroughly juxtaposed when the graft is already divided and transferred to the head (flap in ischemic time). The accuracy of the reconstruction is not high by means of this intraoperative procedure of shaping the graft. Moreover, in cases in which the tumor invades the outer cortex, or when in-continuity resection with facial skin is required, it is then impossible to "precontour" the reconstruction plates as described [12].

More accurate reconstruction planning is possible by means of stereolithographic modeling of the jaw, in which the resection is simulated preoperatively and an acrylic surgical template for reconstruction, which considers dental modeling as well, is manufactured. Pre-contouring and prebending of the reconstruction plate is realizable according to the acrylic surgical template, outside the operation theater; afterward the fixation hardware can be sterilized and is ready for the intervention (Fig. 2). A resected tumor specimen can be helpful for use as a template; however, if the tumor is malignant, most oncologic surgeons would not advocate use of the resected specimen for fear of seeding tumor cells onto the free graft or into the neck [18].

Anesi et al. [19] demonstrated that osteotomies performed using piezosurgical devices show more advanced stages of bone healing compared with rotary instruments. Moreover, even more powerful devices (output power, 75 W) do not alter the process of bone healing. Generally speaking, we recommend piezosurgical devices for improved bone healing, regardless of the chosen fixation system [19–21].

Hidalgo [4] was the first to advocate the use of miniplates (Figs. 8 and 9) and mentioned several advantages, such as ease of application, the low profile of the plates, and superior contour restoration because each osteotomized segment is plated individually. Nevertheless, reconstruction plates also show advantages, e.g., the ease of use of a single plate and the need for fewer screws [4]. Multiple authors have investigated dissimilarities in outcomes between miniplates and reconstruction plates in fibula fixation, without discovering statistically significant differences. Pointing out the comparison of the costs related to different methods, one author reports that several miniplates required for fibula graft-fixing are equivalent to a single reconstruction plate [12].

Following the Hidalgo experience (1989), in the early 2000s, the use of miniplates as opposed to reconstruction plates (lower profiles and smaller screw diameters) has been the subject of intense debate [2, 12, 14, 22].

Fontana et al. [23] and Renderbach et al. [24] reported recently that 2.3 mm locking plates work better with respect to miniplates in an ex vivo study [20, 21]. However, the decision to use miniplates with respect to reconstruction plates remains controversial between the authors, because no significative evidence demonstrates the superiority of one system in jaw reconstruction (Fig. 11) [1, 25, 26].

While in the mandible different authors choose different fixation methods there are more points of agreement in fixation method of the upper jaw reconstruction with fibula flap.

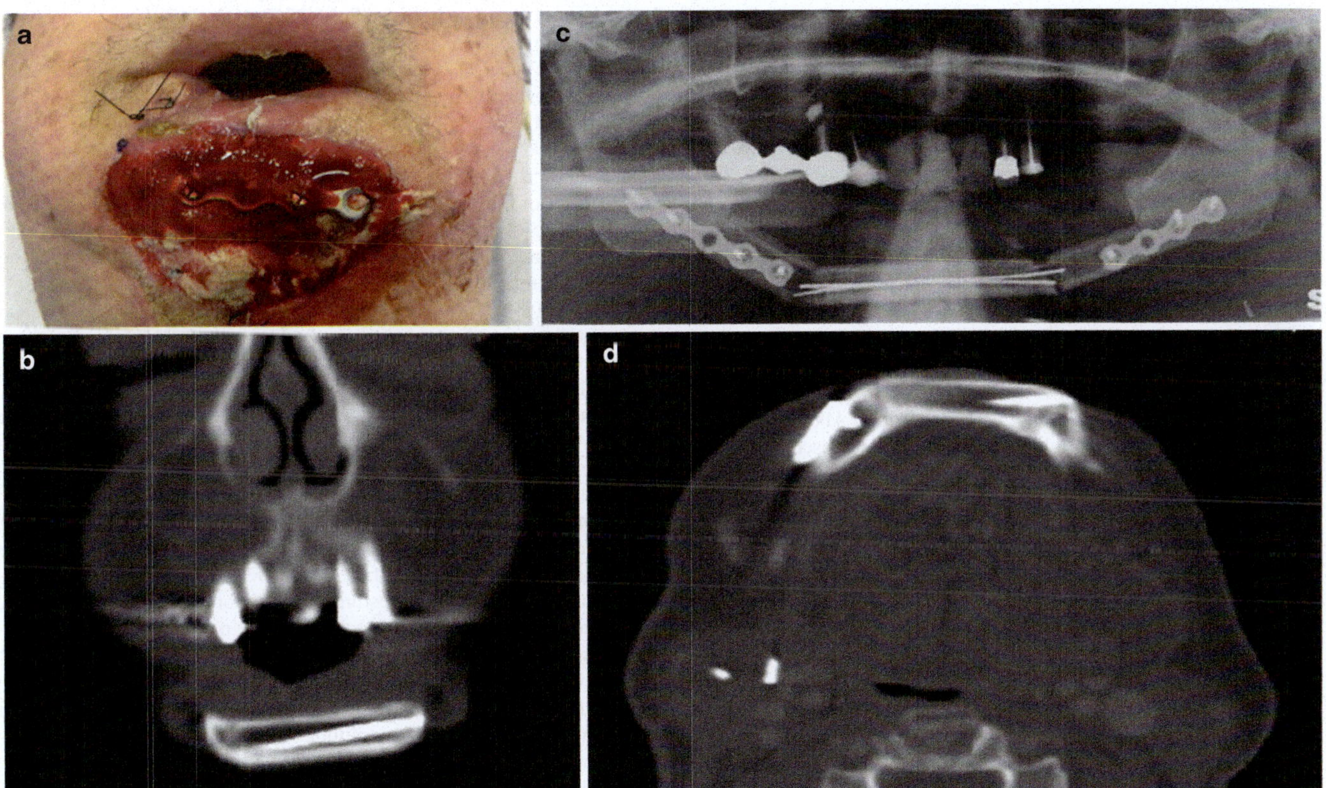

Fig. 11 Reconstruction plate exposure (2.7 mm) after fibula flap for treatment of osteoradionecrosis of the mandible. (**a**) The plate exposure occurred because the quality of the chin skin was poor due to radiation. The first step in healing required removal of the reconstruction plate. (**b**) Since the union period was not complete, the plate was anteriorly cut and removed, while the anterior segment was refixed by a Kirschner wire, less cumbersome compared to reconstruction plate. Here, postoperative orthopantomograph. (**c** and **d**) Postoperative CT scan demonstrated a correct bone union. Afterward a split-thickness skin grafting was performed

Restricted spaces and low load-bearing forces during the union period make miniplates more suitable, in our opinion, with respect to reconstruction bars for fixation in maxilla reconstruction with free fibula flap.

Over the past two decades, the technique has been refined, the applications expanded, and virtual planning for both harvest and inset has been introduced [27].

The accuracy in surgical design tailored to the demands of the patient is increasing thanks to virtual surgical planning. Whereas fibula contouring is digitally planned, miniplates can be easily bent for fibula fixation in virtual planning, one at a time for each osteotomy; though precise, this procedure is time-consuming for multiple osteotomies [1].

Custom-made prebent reconstruction plates are the most recent and the final step of the virtual design process. Reported advantages are a more efficient rate of bony union, improved facial contours, shorter ischemia time, decreased complication rates, and improved patient satisfaction. Fixation of free fibula flap to the natural jaw requires only a few minutes, greatly reducing the total ischemia time [28].

Whereas complications in miniplates and reconstruction plates are similar, the choice of a fixation method for free fibula flap in jaw reconstruction should be tailored to the demands of the defect and patient.

Only custom reconstruction prebent plates prove to be superior to miniplates or to modern reconstruction plates, except for the cost of customized hardware; different health economies limit worldwide accessibility and diffusion of this technology innovation for adding cost [1, 29].

References

1. Al-Bustani S, Austin GK, Ambrose EC, Miller J, Hackman TG, Halvorson EG. Miniplates versus reconstruction bars for oncologic free fibula flap mandible reconstruction. Ann Plast Surg. 2016;77:314–7.
2. Knott PD, Suh JD, Nabili V, Sercarz JA, Head C, Abemayor E, et al. Evaluation of hardware-related complications in vascularized bone grafts with locking mandibular reconstruction plate fixation. Arch Otolaryngol Head Neck Surg. 2007;133:1302–6.
3. Strackee SD, Kroon FH, Bos KE. Fixation methods in mandibular reconstruction using fibula grafts: a comparative study into the relative strength of three different types of osteosynthesis. Head Neck. 2001;23:1–7.
4. Hidalgo DA. Titanium miniplate fixation in free flap mandible reconstruction. Ann Plast Surg. 1989;23:498–507.
5. Boyd JB, Mulholland RS. Fixation of the vascularized bone graft in mandibular reconstruction. Plast Reconstr Surg. 1993;91:274–82.
6. Santamaria E, Wei F-C, Chen HC. Fibula osteoseptocutaneous flap for reconstruction of osteoradionecrosis of the mandible. Plast Reconstr Surg. 1998;101:921–9.
7. Mirante JP, Urken ML, Aviv JE, Brandwein M, Buchbinder D, Biller HF. Resistance to osteoradionecrosis in neovascularised bone. Laryngoscope. 1998;103:1168–73.
8. Capizzi PJ, Jacobsen WM, Meland NB, Smith AA. Lag-screw technique in free osseous mandibular reconstruction. J Reconstr Microsurg. 1998;14:3–10.. discussion 10–1
9. Ellis E 3rd, Ghali GE. Lag screw fixation of anterior mandibular fractures. Oral Maxillofac Surg. 1991;49:13–21.
10. Drugacz J, Lekston Z, Morawiec H, Januszewski K. Use of TiNiCo shape-memory clamps in the surgical treatment of mandibular fractures. J Oral Maxillofac Surg. 1995;53:665–71.
11. Futran ND, Urken ML, Buchbinder D, Moscoso JF, Biller HF. Rigid fixation of vascularized bone grafts in mandibular reconstruction. Arch Otolaryngol Head Neck Surg. 1995;121:70–6.
12. Shaw RJ, Kanatas AN, Lowe D, Brown JS, Rogers SN, Vaughan ED. Comparison of miniplates and reconstruction plates in mandibular reconstruction. Head Neck. 2004;26:456–63.
13. Herford AS, Ellis E 3rd. Use of a locking reconstruction bone plate/screw system for mandibular surgery. J Oral Maxillofac Surg. 1998;56:1261–5.
14. Farwell DG, Kezirian EJ, Heydt JL, Yueh B, Futran ND. Efficacy of small reconstruction plates in vascularized bone graft mandibular reconstruction. Head Neck. 2006;28:573–9.
15. Urken ML, Buchbinder D, Costantino PD, Sinha U, Okay D, Lawson W, et al. Oromandibular reconstruction using microvascular composite flaps: Report of 210 cases. Arch Otolaryngol Head Neck Surg. 1998;124:46–55.
16. Schmelzeisen R, Rahn BA, Brennwald J. Fixation of vascularised bone grafts. J Craniomaxillofac Surg. 1993;21:113–9.
17. Ung F, Rocco JW, Deschler DG. Temporary intraoperative external fixation in mandibular reconstruction. Laryngoscope. 2002;112:1569–73.
18. Ostric SA, Martin WJ, Stock C, Bittar SM. The model graft: reconstruction of the maxilla using a fibular bone graft template. J Craniofac Surg. 2006;17(1):145–7.
19. Anesi A, Ferretti M, Cavani F, Salvatori R, Bianchi M, Russo A, et al. Structural and ultrastructural analyses of bone regeneration in rabbit cranial osteotomy: Piezosurgery versus traditional osteotomes. J Craniomaxillofac Surg. 2018;46(1):107–18.
20. Chiarini L, Albanese M, Anesi A, Galzignato PF, Mortellaro C, Nocini P, et al. Surgical treatment of unilateral condylar hyperplasia with piezosurgery. J Craniofac Surg. 2014;25:808–10.
21. Turra M, Bertossi D, Bissolotti G, Anesi A, Chiarini L, Nocini PF. O.095 Genioplasty with piezosurgery. J Craniomaxillofac Surg. 2008;36:S24. https://doi.org/10.1016/S1010-5182(08)71219-8.
22. Militsakh ON, Wallace DI, Kriet JD, Girod DA, Olvera MS, Tsue TT. Use of the 2.0-mm locking reconstruction plate in oromandibular reconstruction after composite resection. Otolaryngol Head Neck Surg. 2004;131(5):660–5.
23. Fontana SC, Smith RB, Nazir N, Andrews BT. Biomechanical assessment of fixation methods for segmental mandible reconstruction with fibula in the polyurethane model. Microsurgery. 2016;36:330–3.
24. Rendenbach C, Kohlmeier C, Suling A, Assaf AT, Catala-Lehnen P, Amling M, et al. Prospective biomechanical analysis of donor-site morbidity after fibula free flap. J Craniomaxillofac Surg. 2016;44:155–9.
25. Schupp W, Arzdorf M, Linke B, Gutwald R. Biomechanical testing of different osteosynthesis systems for segmental resection of the mandible. J Oral Maxillofac Surg. 2007;65:924–30.
26. Trainotti S, Raith S, Kesting M, Eichhorn S, Bauer F, Kolk A, et al. Locking versus nonlocking plates in mandibular reconstruction with fibular graft–a biomechanical ex vivo study. Clin Oral Investig. 2014;18:1291–8.
27. Antony AK, Chen WF, Kolokythas A, Weimer KA, Cohen MN. Use of virtual surgery and stereolithography-guided osteotomy for mandibular reconstruction with the free fibula. Plast Reconstr Surg. 2011;128:1080–4.
28. Cornelius CP, Smolka W, Giessler GA, Wilde F, Probst FA. Patient-specific reconstruction plates are the missing link in computer-assisted mandibular reconstruction: a showcase for technical description. J Craniomaxillofac Surg. 2015;43(5):624–9.
29. Arce K, Waris S, Alexander AE, Ettinger KS. Novel patient-specific 3-dimensional printed fixation tray for mandibular reconstruction with fibular free flaps. J Oral Maxillofac Surg. 2018;76(10):2211–9.

Part V

Endosseous Dental Implants

Technique

Luigi Chiarini, Alexandre Anesi, and Sara Negrello

The loss of teeth and of the alveolar and basal jaw bone can lead to significant impairment of mastication. Severe mandibular or maxillary bone defects due to surgical ablation of tumors, congenital malformations, atrophy, trauma injury, osteomyelitis, or osteoradionecrosis may lead to aesthetic and functional deficit, such as facial contour disfigurement, loss of lip support, malocclusion, and impaired functions of speech, swallowing, and saliva retention [1].

The aim of maxillary or mandibular reconstruction must be to restore not only aesthetics but also complete oral function [2].

Cortical bone thickness, height, and bicortical structure of the fibula shaft are ideal for long-term implant-borne prosthetic rehabilitation. Fibular cortical thickness is superior with respect to the iliac crest or the scapula crest [3–5].

However, a vascularized mono-barrel fibula flap does not provide an adequate basis for prosthetic rehabilitation. It lacks sufficient bone height to restore both the mandibular skeletal base and the alveolar ridge, and the thickness of its soft tissues and the absence of a pelvi-lingual/vestibular groove complicate dental prosthesis retention [6].

The possibility of placing endosseous dental implants in the reconstructed areas with the fibula permits us to overcome the problems related to dental rehabilitation with removable prostheses [7].

The efficacy of dental implants placed into free fibula flaps for orofacial reconstruction has been thoroughly proved [1, 8].

Some authors have reported the possibility of inserting implants into the free fibula flap during the primary reconstruction, because at that point there is better access to the bone, interdental relationships are easier to determine, and oral rehabilitation can be attained in a shorter period of time.

There are several disadvantages, however, that may result from this rehabilitative choice: endosseous dental implant placement procedure is time-consuming; the preoperative planning becomes complicated; implants can be entirely lost in the case of flap failure.

The major disadvantage of immediate implant insertion concerns the high possibility of misalignment of the fixtures. Gross alterations in the anatomical situation and/or in the intermaxillary relationship occur after ablative surgery, in segmental mandibular resections in particular. Improperly positioned implants impair the prosthodontic treatment and in some cases may not even be used in the final prosthodontic rehabilitation of the patient.

Other disadvantages include the risk of interference with or delay of oncological therapy, especially of postoperative irradiation. Mucosal lesions and implant exposure are postoperative treatment complications associated with implantation performed at the same time as ablative surgery. Moreover, a prosthesis cannot be realistically provided until the oral soft tissues have returned to a healthy state [3, 9–12].

In delayed implant borne-prosthetic rehabilitation (a few years after the fibula graft), planning accurate evaluation for unknown administration of bisphosphonate or other antiresorptive drug treatment should be made, in order to avoid medication-related osteonecrosis of the jaw (MRONJ) and antiresorptive drug-related osteonecrosis of the jaw (ARONJ) [13]. The use of oral implants in irradiated tissue is not considered to be contraindicated, although it has been reported that the risk of implant failure increases with losses up to 35% (mean 13.6%, range 0–36%), while in non-irradiated mandibles the implant survival rate is 90% (mean 96.1%, range 74.8–100%) in most studies [14].

The timing of the implantation procedure, with regard to the effects of irradiation on the jawbone, remains inconclusive for lack of scientific evidence. Typically, dental implants are placed 6 months after radiation therapy [15].

L. Chiarini (✉) · A. Anesi · S. Negrello
Cranio-Maxillo-Facial Surgery Unit, University Hospital of Modena, Modena, Italy
e-mail: luigi.chiarini@unimore.it; alexandre.anesi@unimore.it

G. De Santis et al. (eds.), *Atlas of Mandibular and Maxillary Reconstruction with the Fibula Flap*,
https://doi.org/10.1007/978-3-030-10684-3_11

There are reports about an improvement in the bone healing capacity over a 12-month period following irradiation, while others report a continuously progressive loss of capillaries in the mandible following irradiation [16].

Other authors recommend implant insertion in a "window" between 1 and 6 months after radiation therapy. In this period, the early effects of radiation are resolved and long-term vascular changes (progressive endarteritis) associated with radiation treatment may not have taken place. Also, the bone is still relatively well vascularized. In oncologic patients, we must also consider potential tumor recurrence [17, 18]. Claudy and coworkers recently published a systematic review in which higher risk of failure may occur if endosseous dental implants are placed within 12 months of radiation therapy [19].

The fibula flap, moreover, can modify its morphology and assume the characteristics of the native bone. Therefore, a 6-month delay before implantation is safer in non-irradiated patients (Figs. 1 and 2) [4, 21, 22].

Osseointegrated dental implant placement typically requires a two-stage procedure. The first stage is planned on postoperative investigations and is performed 6 months after the primary surgery to allow complete bone union between the fibula and the native bone. Plates and screws are usually removed in the first-stage implant surgery. The second stage consists of implant exposure and vestibuloplasty 9 months after ablative surgery, and after an additional 3 months, the implant-supported prosthesis may be completed.

An orthopantomograph should be taken at 6 months to assess the healing of bone segments. CT images are important to understand the bone volume and quality so that the number, axis, and size of implants can be ascertained and chosen. The dimensions of endosseous implants depend on the size of the bone (fibula height) and generally do not exceed 13 mm in height and 3.5–4.5 mm in diameter.

Piezoelectric surgery could be considered a reliable and safe alternative to conventional drill technique for dental endosseous implant site preparation [23]. Anesi et al. [24] demonstrated that osteotomies performed using piezosurgical devices show more advanced stages of bone healing compared with rotary instruments. Moreover, even more

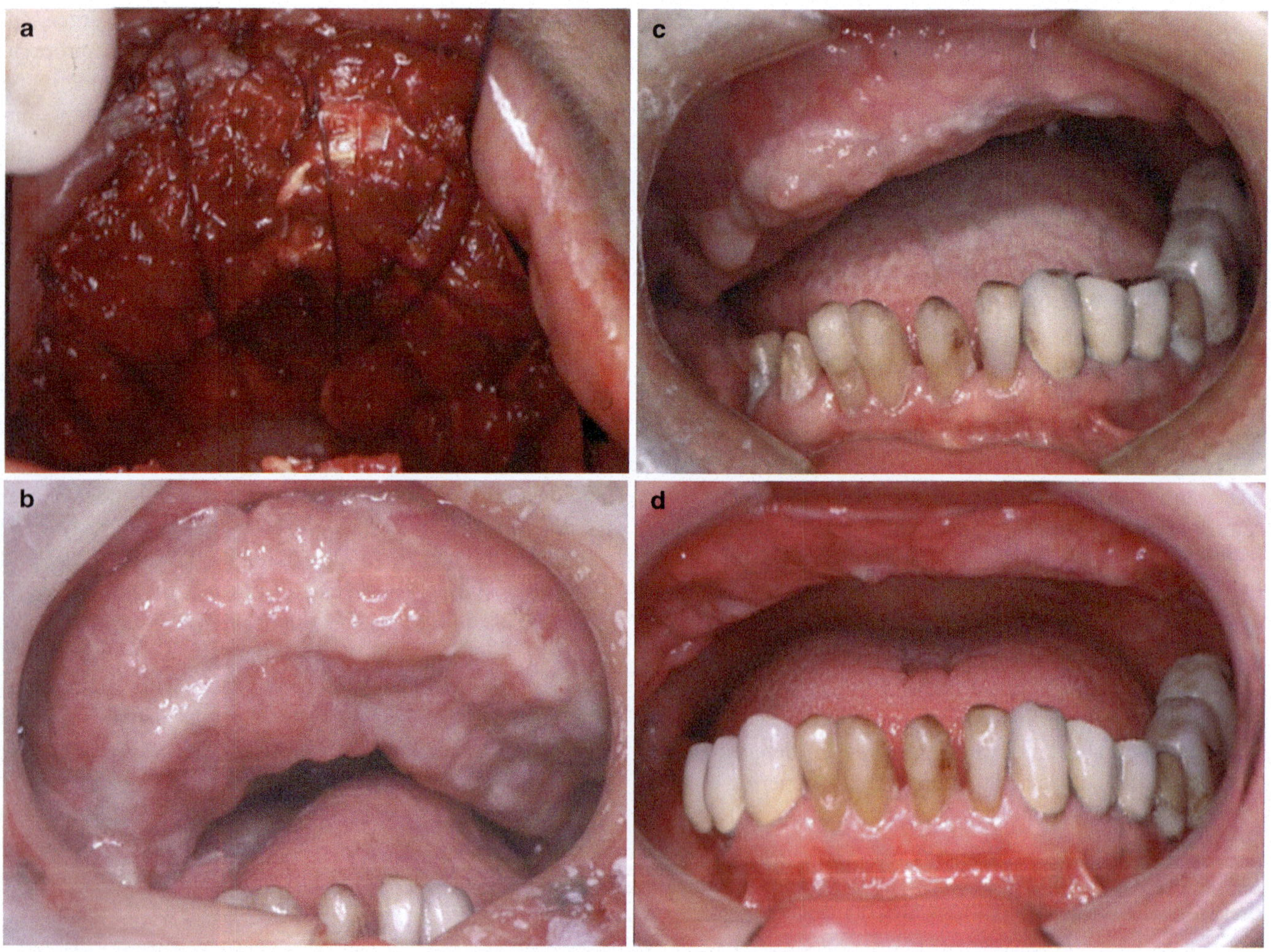

Fig. 1 Healing process of myosseous free fibula flap to restore alveolar ridge. (**a**) Operative view after fibula insetting; a thin cuff of muscle is left directly exposed in oral cavity. (**b**) 1–3 weeks of healing. (**c**) 4–6 weeks of healing. (**d**) 6 months of healing [20]

Fig. 2 Spontaneous fibula remodeling 6 months after the intervention. (**a**) The fibula flap contoured by wedge osteotomy technique and fixed to native maxilla. (**b**) The reconstructed alveolar process, like the native one, is horseshoe-shaped

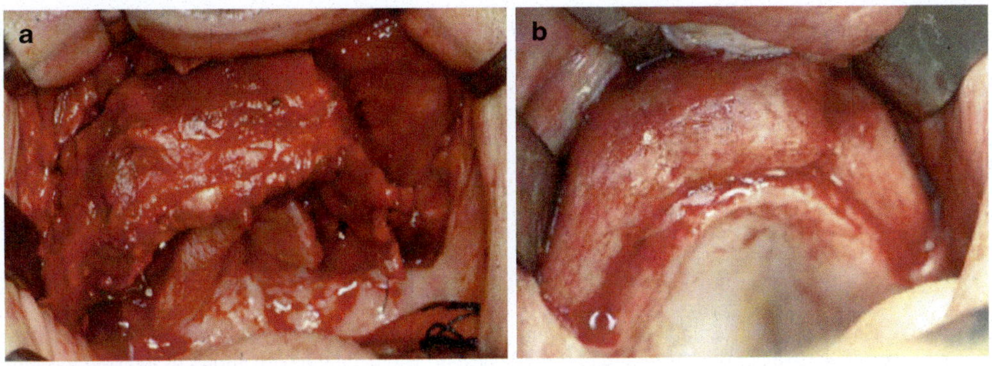

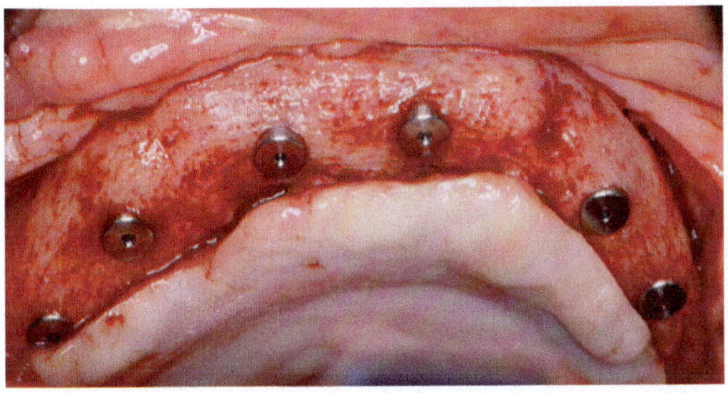

Fig. 3 Delayed implant placement on a fibular free flap, 6 months after the intervention [4, 22, 26, 28, 29]

powerful devices (output power of 75 W) do not alter the process of bone healing [24, 25]. Some authors have proposed a flapless approach as being less traumatic for the tissues. In the literature, some works support the navigation system for implant placement [26, 27].

In surgical planning it is useful to place the pedicle under the flap to avoid damage to the vascularization of the flap during implant surgery. An incision is made through soft tissues to an accurate exposition of the fibular bone. As stated above, reconstructive plates or miniplates are usually removed at the same time as implant placement (Fig. 3). Complete closure of the implantation site is necessary to prevent infection. A 7-day course of antibiotic therapy is given as closure and healing of the soft tissues occurs. The sutures are removed 15 days after surgery. Radiological and clinical follow-up is scheduled immediately after surgery and 1 month after surgery and then before the second stage of the procedure.

A recurrent problem in prosthetic planning is the vertical discrepancy between the fibula flap and the native bone, particularly in patients treated by segmental resection of the mandible and having residual dentition on the healthy side [1]. A solution might be to rebuild the prosthesis to conform to over-dimensioned teeth; however, aggravated oral hygiene, recurrent soft-tissue infection, and poor dental aesthetics are foreseeable consequences.

Various techniques for vertical bone augmentation in fibula flap are reported in the literature and are described in chapters "Bone Augmentation" and "Second Vascularized Fibula Flap and Osteotomy to Correct Malocclusion".

Depending on local healing, the second stage of implant surgery can be started between 3 and 6 months after implant placement, in compliance with the Brånemark protocol. The implants are uncovered, tested for stability (see chapter "Assessment"), and fitted with the transmucosal abutments. Most of the time, a vestibuloplasty can be performed at this time, sometimes associated with epithelial graft, to create a larger prosthetic space and to increase mobility of the lower lip and cheek.

The fibula flap is commonly harvested as osteocutaneous flap, so that a skin paddle is harvested with the fibula bone graft. The skin paddle is bulky, much thicker than the gingiva, not fixed to the bone by the periosteum, and not keratinized. Oral rehabilitation is limited by excessive thickness and mobility of the overlying skin and soft tissues and obliteration of the vestibule, because these anatomical and morphological factors generally lead to poor hygiene around implants. Hyperplastic peri-implant tissue, pocket formation, soft-tissue infections, and recurrent abscesses that start as peri-implant marginal bone loss may eventually lead to failure of the implant and of the dental rehabilitation [30]. In oncologic defects, the skin paddle in the fibula transplant is usually not optimal for peri-implant coverage. Hence constant assessment and monitoring of peri-implant hard- and soft-tissue parameters are extremely important in evaluating the performance of implant-supported treatment in reconstructed jaws [1].

Thinning of the skin flap and vestibuloplasty are often required [31].

Several techniques are used in soft-tissue management after a fibula vascularized graft, such as skin graft, mucosa graft, or biological membranes (Figs. 4–7).

The osteo-periosteal flap is of considerable utility to avoid these complications. Unfortunately the osteo-periosteal flap of the fibula is not suitable in the case of oral malignant tumors, in which resection of large areas of soft tissue and mucosa is needed: the skin paddle becomes inevitable [34–36].

An osteo-periosteal flap may be easily used in rehabilitation for severe atrophies or in tumors confined to the bone tissue with little resection of the mucosa.

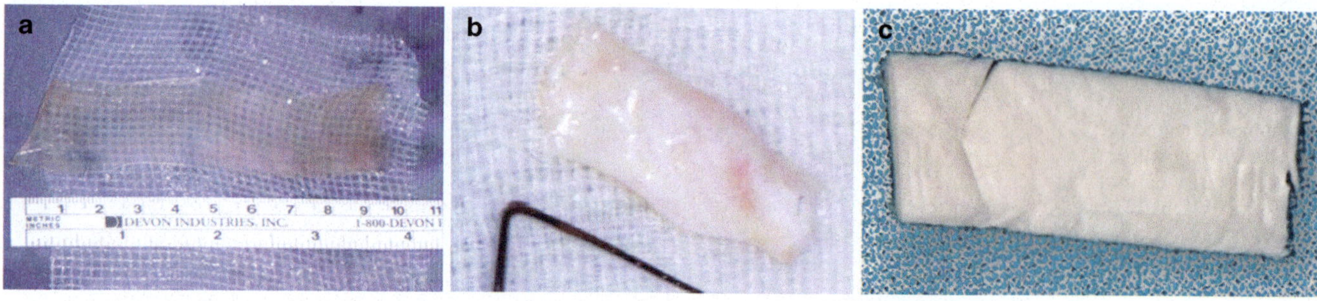

Fig. 4 We usually perform vestibuloplasty 9 months after bone reconstruction. (**a**) Split-thickness skin grafts are used for large defects and palatal fibrous-connective tissue grafts (**b**) are used for mild ones. (**c**) Biomembrane use allows us to avoid morbidity

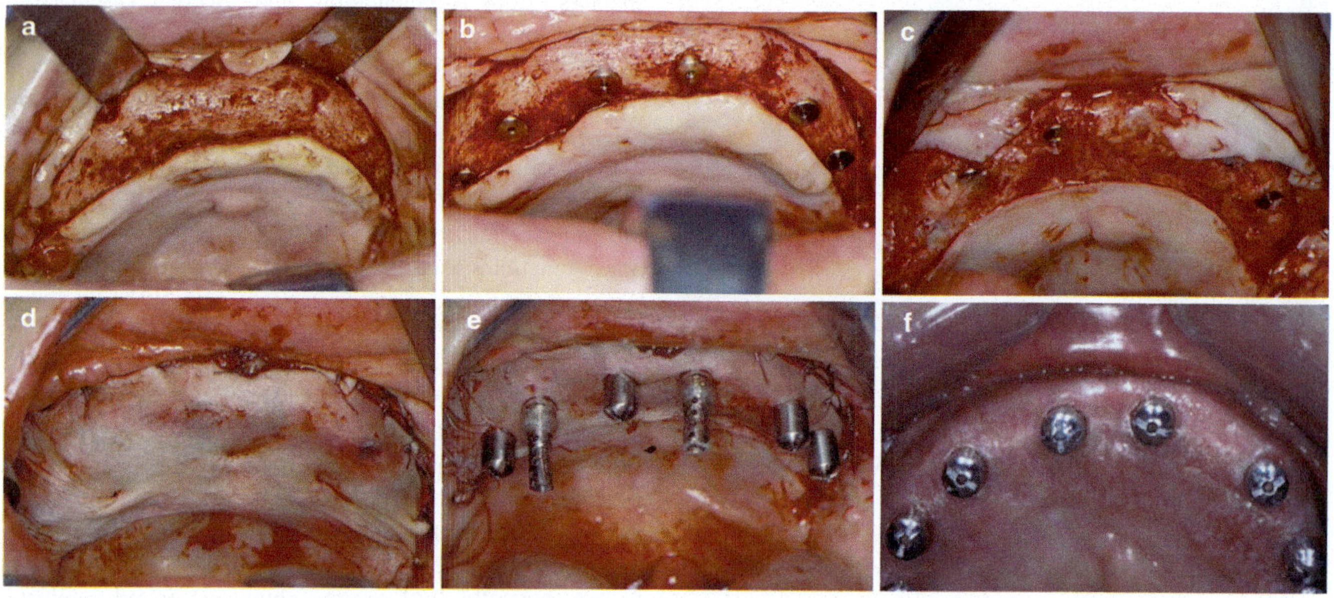

Fig. 5 Vestibuloplasty and split-thickness skin graft onto a fibula flap for upper jaw restoration. (**a**) An incision is made through soft tissues to an accurate exposition of the fibular bone. (**b**) Endosseous dental implant placement. (**c**) Superior vestibular groove repositioning for vestibule-sulcoplasty. (**d**) Split-thickness skin grafting of restored alveolar crest. (**e**) The implants are uncovered, tested for stability, and fitted with the transmucosal abutments. (**f**) Healed peri-implant soft tissues

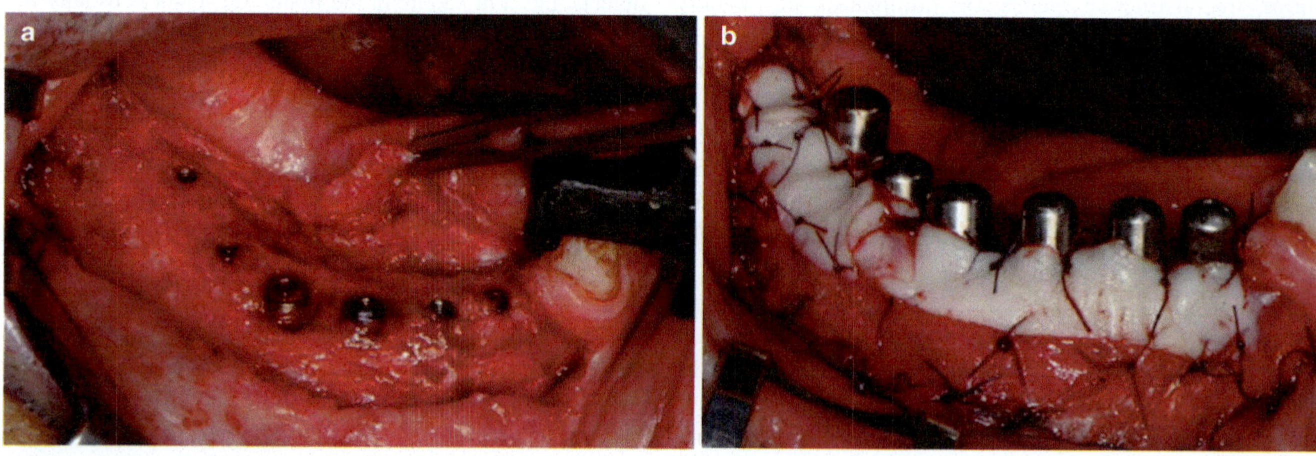

Fig. 6 Vestibuloplasty and palatal fibrous-connective tissue graft onto a fibula flap for mandible restoration. (**a**) The implants are uncovered. (**b**) Palatal fibrous-connective tissue grafting. (**c**) Surgical dressing and periodontal pack. (**d**) Healed peri-implant soft tissues [32]

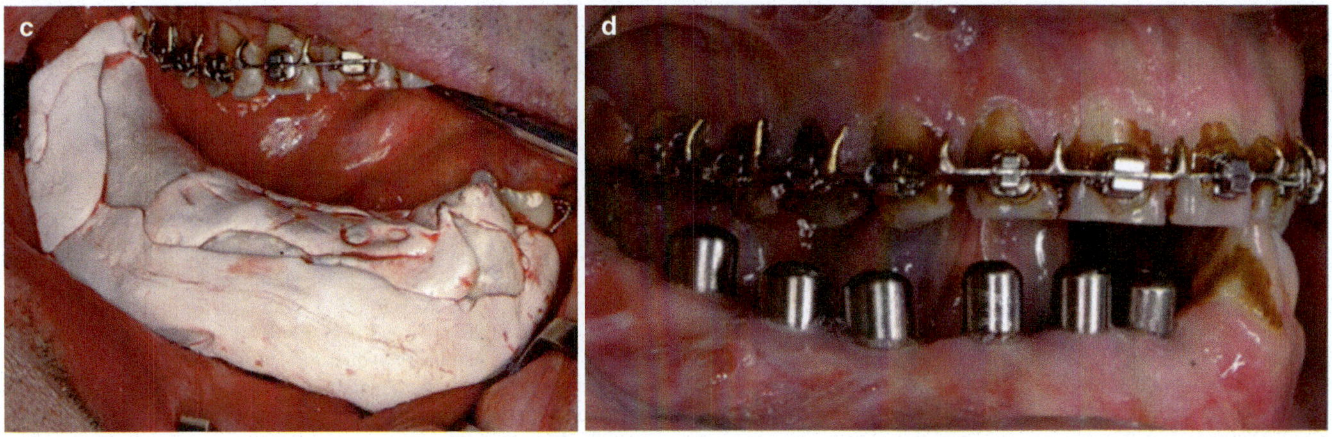

Fig. 6 (continued)

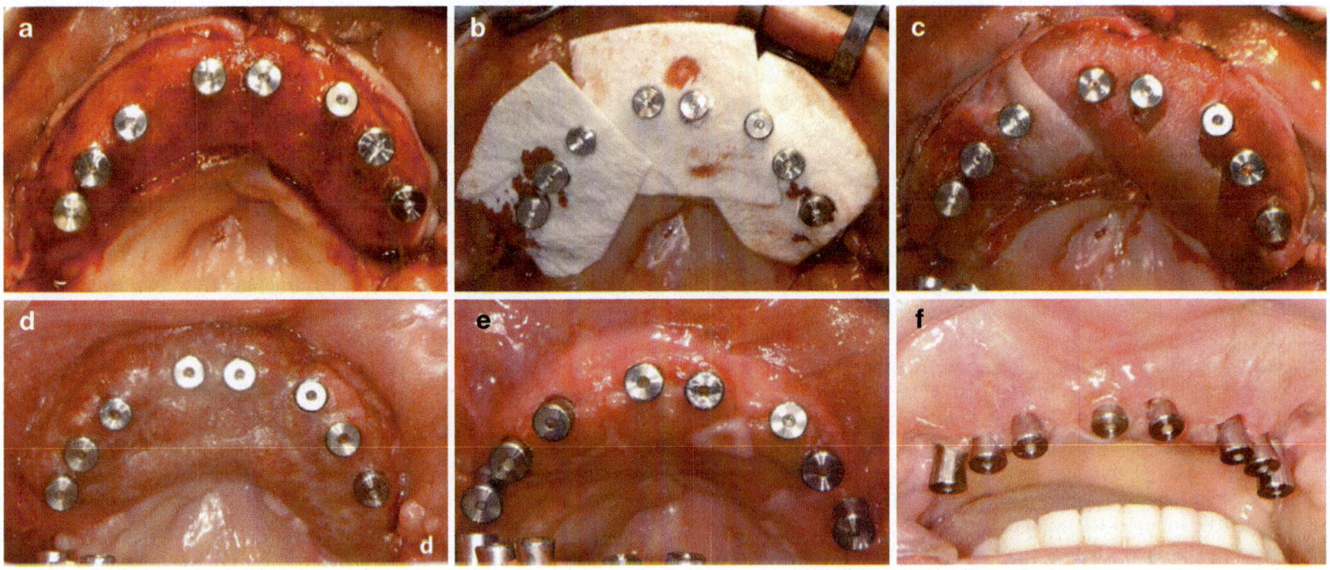

Fig. 7 Vestibuloplasty and biomembrane (three-dimensional collagen tissue matrix derived of porcine dermis) placement onto a fibula flap for mandible restoration. (**a**) Split-thickness flap sutured on the vestibule to prepare the surgical bed for membrane placement (**b**) Positioning of membrane on the prepared bed. (**c**) Oral appearance at the end of membrane placing. (**d**) Healing at 14 days after surgery. (**e**) Healing at 30 days after surgery. (**f**) Healing at 2 months after surgery. Deepening of the vestibule is well maintained [33]

References

1. Chiapasco M, Biglioli F, Autelitano L, Romeo E, Brusati R. Clinical outcome of dental implants placed in fibula-free flaps used for the reconstruction of maxillo-mandibular defects following ablation for tumors or osteoradionecrosis. Clin Oral Implants Res. 2006;17(2):220–8.
2. Hidalgo DA. Fibula free flap: a new method of mandible reconstruction. Plast Reconstr Surg. 1989;84(1):71–9.
3. Hayter JP, Cawood JI. Oral rehabilitation with endosteal implants and free flaps. Int J Oral Maxillofac Surg. 1996;25:3–12.
4. Moscoso JF, Keller J, Genden E, Weinberg H, Biller HF, Buchbinder D, et al. Vascularized bone flaps in oromandibular reconstruction. A comparative anatomic study of bone stock from various donor sites to assess suitability for endosseous dental implants. Arch Otolaryngol Head Neck Surg. 1994;120:36–43.
5. Chang YM, Santamaria E, Wei FC, Chen HC, Chan CP, Shen YF, et al. Primary insertion of osseointegrated dental implants into fibula osteoseptocutaneous free flap for mandible reconstruction. Plast Reconstr Surg. 1998;102:680–8.
6. Bedogni A, Anesi A, Fior A, Bettini G, Nocini PF. Microsurgical reconstruction of the mandible in a patient with Evans syndrome: a case report and review of the literature. J Reconstr Microsurg. 2013;29(8):545–50. https://doi.org/10.1055/s-0033-1348898.
7. Smolka K, Kraehenbuehl M, Eggensperger N, Hallermann W, Thoren H, Iizuka T, et al. Fibula free flap reconstruction of the mandible in cancer patients: evaluation of a combined surgical and prosthodontic treatment concept. Oral Oncol. 2008;44(6):571–81.
8. Bertossi D, Bissolotti G, Corrocher G, Anesi A, Nocini PF. O.301 The use of tapered dental implants in severe jaw atrophies. J Craniomaxillofac Surg. 2008;36(Suppl 1):S76. https://doi.org/10.1016/S1010-5182(08)71425-2.

9. Garrett N, Roumanas ED, Blackwell KE, Freymiller E, Abemayor E, Wong WK, et al. Efficacy of conventional and implant-supported mandibular resection prostheses: study overview and treatment outcomes. J Prosthet Dent. 2006;96:13–24.
10. Chang YM, Wallace CG, Tsai CY, Shen YF, Hsu YM, Wei FC. Dental implant outcome after primary implantation into double barreled fibula osteoseptocutaneous free flap-reconstructed mandible. Plast Reconstr Surg. 2011;128:1220–8.
11. Rohner D, Bucher P, Kunz C, Hammer B, Schenk RK, Prein J. Treatment of severe atrophy of the maxilla with the prefabricated free vascularized fibula flap. Clin Oral Implants Res. 2002;13:44–52.
12. Roumanas ED, Garrett N, Blackwell KE, Freymiller E, Abemayor E, Wong WK, et al. Masticatory and swallowing threshold performances with conventional and implant-supported prostheses after mandibular fibula free-flap reconstruction. J Prosthet Dent. 2006;96(4):289–97.
13. Pozzi S, Anesi A, Generali L, Bari A, Consolo U, Chiarini L. Bisphosphonate-related osteonecrosis of the jaw (BRONJ). In: Tsesis I, editor. Complications in endodontic surgery: prevention, identification and management. 1. New York, NY: Springer; 2014. p. 153–165. doi:https://doi.org/10.1007/978-3-642-54218-3. ISBN 978-3-642-54217-6; ISBN 978-3-642-54218-3 (eBook).
14. Hundepool AC, Dumans AG, Hofer SO, Fokkens NJ, Rayat SS, van der Meij EH, et al. Rehabilitation after mandibular reconstruction with fibula free-flap: clinical outcome and quality of life assessment. Int J Oral Maxillofac Surg. 2008;37(11):1009–13.
15. Batenburg RH, Meijer HJ, Raghoebar GM, Vissink A. Treatment concept for mandibular overdentures supported by endosseous implants: a literature review. Int J Oral Maxillofac Implants. 1998;13(4):539–45.
16. Javed F, Al-Hezaimi K, Al-Rasheed A, Almas K, Romanos GE. Implant survival rate after oral cancer therapy: a review. Oral Oncol. 2010;46:854–9.
17. Jacobsson M, Tjellström A, Thomsen P, Albrektsson T, Turesson I. Integration of implants in irradiated bone. Histologic and clinical study. Ann Otol Rhinol Laryngol. 1988;97:337–40.
18. Granström G, Bergström K, Tjellström A, Brånemark PI. A detailed study of titanium implants lost in irradiated tissues. Int J Oral Maxillofac Implants. 1994;9(6):653–62.
19. Marx RE, Johnson RP. Studies in the radiobiology of osteoradionecrosis and their clinical significance. Oral Surg Oral Med Oral Pathol. 1987;64(4):379–90.
20. Elshal EE, Inokuchi T, Sekine J, Sano K. Experimental study of epithelialization of the muscle-only flap in the oral cavity. J Oral Maxillofac Surg. 1997;55(12):1423–30.. discussion 1431–2
21. Claudy MP, Miguens SA Jr, Celeste RK, Camara Parente R, Hernandez PA, da Silva AN Jr. Time interval after radiotherapy and dental implant failure: systematic review of observational studies and meta-analysis. Clin Implant Dent Relat Res. 2015;17:402–11.
22. Roumanas ED, Markowitz BL, Lorant JA, Calcaterra TC, Jones NF, Beumer J 3rd. Reconstructed mandibular defects: fibula free flaps and osseointegrated implants. Plast Reconstr Surg. 1997;99(2):356–65.
23. Atieh MA, Alsabeeha NHM, Tawse-Smith A, Duncan WJ. Piezoelectric versus conventional implant site preparation: a systematic review and metaanalysis. Clin Implant Dent Relat Res. 2018;20:261–70.
24. Anesi A, Ferretti M, Cavani F, Salvatori R, Bianchi M, Russo A, Chiarini L, Palumbo C. Structural and ultrastructural analyses of bone regeneration in rabbit cranial osteotomy: piezosurgery versus traditional osteotomes. J Craniomaxillofac Surg. 2018;46(1):107–18. https://doi.org/10.1016/j.jcms.2017.10.004.
25. Chiarini L, Albanese M, Anesi A, Galzignato PF, Mortellaro C, Nocini PF, Bertossi D. Surgical treatment of unilateral condylar hyperplasia with piezosurgery. J Craniofac Surg. 2014;25(3):808–10. https://doi.org/10.1097/SCS.0000000000000699.
26. De Santis G, Nocini PF, Chiarini L, Bedogni A. Functional rehabilitation of the atrophic mandible and maxilla with fibula flaps and implant-supported prosthesis. Plast Reconstr Surg. 2004;113(1):88–98.. discussion 99–100
27. Horowitz A, Orentlicher G, Goldsmith D. Computerized implantology for the irradiated patient. J Oral Maxillofac Surg. 2009;67(3):619–23.
28. Gurlek A, Miller MJ, Jacob RF, Lively JA, Schusterman MA. Functional results of dental restoration with osseointegrated implants after mandible reconstruction. Plast Reconstr Surg. 1998;101(3):650–5.. discussion 656–9
29. De Santis G, Chiarini L, Bedogni A, Nocini PF. Jaw reconstruction by free fibular transfer: emphasis on osseointegrated implants, TMJ and maxilla reconstruction. Eur J Plast Surg. 1999;22:62–8.
30. Albanese M, Aquilini S, Toller N, Bertossi D, Corrocher G, Anesi A, Nocini PF. O.319 Gingival hyperplasia and PAI-1: a case report. J Craniomaxillofac Surg. 2008;36(Suppl1):S80. https://doi.org/10.1016/S1010-5182(08)71443-4.
31. Bell RB, Weimer KA, Dierks EJ, Buehler M, Lubek JE. Computer planning and intraoperative navigation for palatomaxillary and mandibular reconstruction with fibular free flaps. J Oral Maxillofac Surg. 2011;69(3):724–32.
32. Chang YM, Chan CP, Shen YF, Wei FC. Soft tissue management using palatal mucosa around endosteal implants in vascularized composite grafts in the mandible. Int J Oral Maxillofac Surg. 1999;28(5):341–3.
33. Nocini PF, Castellani R, Zanotti G, Gelpi F, Covani U, Marconcini S, de Santis D. Extensive keratinized tissue augmentation during implant rehabilitation after Le Fort I osteotomy: using a new porcine collagen membrane (Mucoderm). J Craniofac Surg. 2014;25(3):799–803.
34. Hakim SG, Driemel O, Jacobsen HC, Hermes D, Sieg P. Exposure of implants using a modified multiple-flap transposition vestibuloplasty. Br J Oral Maxillofac Surg. 2006;44(6):507–10.
35. Deganello A, Gitti G, Parrinello G, Muratori E, Larotonda G, Gallo O. Cost analysis in oral cavity and oropharyngeal reconstructions with microvascular and pedicled flaps. Acta Otorhinolaryngol Ital. 2013;33(6):380–7.
36. Salvatori P, Paradisi S, Calabrese L, Zani A, Cantù G, Cappiello J, et al. Patients' survival after free flap reconstructive surgery of head and neck squamous cell carcinoma: a retrospective multicentre study. Acta Otorhinolaryngol Ital. 2014;34(2):99–104.

Assessment

Alexandre Anesi, Sara Negrello, and Luigi Chiarini

Introduction

In order to achieve an adequate oral rehabilitation after reconstruction of the jaw, a consistent prosthetic treatment is necessary [1].

Placement of dental implants represents the most successful treatment modality of rehabilitation in the reconstructed jaw, whether with revascularized fibula or iliac crest flap.

However, implant failure rates are in the range of 5–8% for routine procedures and up to 20% in major grafting cases during at least 5 years of function [2].

Identified risk factors for implant loss are (1) low primary implant stability, (2) low bone density, (3) short implants, and (4) overload [3]. Therefore, a sure implant stability is a determinant for a successful clinical outcome with dental implants.

The main determinants of implant stability are the mechanical properties of the bone tissue at the implant site, and how the contact between the implant neck and the cortical bone plate is achieved [4]. If we presume a correct surgical technique and a good implant design, the bone density determines the primary implant stability at the time of surgery [5] Piezoelectric surgery could be considered a reliable and safe alternative to conventional drill technique for dental endosseous implant site preparation [6]. Anesi et al. (2018) demonstrated that osteotomies performed using piezosurgical devices show more advanced stages of bone healing compared with rotary instruments. Moreover, even more powerful devices (output power of 75 W) do not alter the process of bone healing [7].

A stable implant can exhibit different degrees of displacement or resistance to load, which corresponds to varying degrees of stability. Conversely, a failed implant shows clinical mobility on the macroscale, as the implant is surrounded by a fibrous scar tissue [4]. An increasing degree of micro-mobility is present until clinical failure of the implant.

This suggests that techniques to measure and to monitor implant micro-motion/stability could give the clinician the opportunity to optimize implant treatment (i.e., increase the stability at placement, time before loading, follow-up of stability after a period of loading). Insertion torque, Periotest, and resonance frequency analysis suitable to measure primary implant stability.

Nevertheless, the resonance frequency analysis is the only method that can detect variations in different bone densities, which may be measured even during the follow-up of the implant [8].

Some 20 years ago, Meredith and coworkers [9] developed resonance frequency analysis (RFA) for implant stability measurements, a technique which today is commercially available as Osstell (Osstell AB, Gothenburg, Sweden) and more recently as PenguinRFA (Integration Diagnostics Sweden AB, Gothenburg, Sweden) (Fig. 1).

Recent in vitro works have confirmed the RFA technique to correlate with implant micromobility/displacement, which in turn is mainly determined by the bone density [10, 11].

Bone density is a major determinant of RFA measurement, as shown in numerous studies, and correlates with insertion torque measurements and with quantitative CT [12–14]. A new unit called implant stability quotient (ISQ) was established. The ISQ scale runs from 1 to 100 units, where the former is the lowest and the latter the highest degree of stability.

Fig. 1 PenguinRFA Instrument (Integration Diagnostics Sweden AB, Gothenburg, Sweden)

A. Anesi (✉) · S. Negrello · L. Chiarini
Cranio-Maxillo-Facial Surgery Unit, University Hospital of Modena, Modena, Italy
e-mail: alexandre.anesi@unimore.it; luigi.chiarini@unimore.it

G. De Santis et al. (eds.), *Atlas of Mandibular and Maxillary Reconstruction with the Fibula Flap*,
https://doi.org/10.1007/978-3-030-10684-3_12

Proposed Interpretations of RFA Measurements

In the authors' opinion, Sennerby and Meredith provided simple operative suggestions for clinical decision-making during implant treatment and follow-up with regard to healing times, loading protocol, and identification of implants at risk for failure [4]. The ISQ measurements have been considered strictly interconnected with clinical/radiographic findings.

It seems that implants with low and/or falling ISQ values pose an increased risk for failure when compared to implants with high and/or increasing values.

With follow-up measurements, the changes of stability can be registered, and repeated measures can be taken in case of low or falling values, i.e., prolonged healing and unloading. We can consider "safe" those implants showing primary ISQ values of 70 and above. The health state of implant-bone interface might be "questionable" with an ISQ value below, for instance, 55. An intermediate group is represented by implants with an ISQ from 55 to 70. The implants showing primary ISQ values of 70 and above may be suitable for immediate loading protocols, while a healing period is useful for implants with an ISQ from 55 to 70. In the group of implants with an ISQ below 55, a second measurement after healing will confirm that an increased stability has been achieved. If low ISQ values are still obtained after an initial healing period, the implant may be left for further healing. For implants with very low ISQ values (<55, the red zone), measures to improve stability should be considered, such as by immediately replacing the implant with a longer, wider, and/or tapered implant, prolonging the healing period, and checking stability.

Falling ISQ values after some time of loading, particularly in immediate/early loading, may be an unfavorable reaction to loading.

Consideration should be given to making a check of occlusion or unloading with a period of healing until the ISQ value has caught up. Moreover, since the ISQ technique is sensitive to crestal bone loss and reduces the ISQ level with 2–3 units/mm, this should be controlled with an intraoral radiograph.

RFA Measurements and Free Revascularized Bone Flaps

Möehlhenrich et al. measured the primary and secondary stability of the implants in patients who had reconstructions of the jaw by revascularized free flaps either from the fibula or iliac crest [15].

Microvascular bone grafts result in low bone resorption rates, independent of their origin in the early healing period, with respect to non-revascularized bone grafts [16].

The fibular flap is commonly used for jaw reconstruction.

A large amount of bone is provided by the microvascular iliac crest bone flap: the greater height of the bony flap allows for a reconstruction similar to the native jaw morphology. Therefore, adequate implant placement without additional bone augmentation can be achieved with microvascular iliac crest flap, due to the acceptable implant-to-crown ratio.

For long-term stability, peri-implant bone and soft tissues are the major determinants. In oncologic defects, the soft tissues by the skin paddle in the fibula graft are usually not optimal for peri-implant coverage.

Previous ex vivo investigation of human bone demonstrated that stabilized implants in fibula flap presented significantly higher primary stability values with respect to iliac crest or scapula bone. This is owing to the higher proportion of cortical to cancellous bone in fibula flap. These findings are related to the contact between the implant neck and the cortical bone plate, which increases the primary stability of the implant [17].

The results of Moehlhenrich's [15] in vivo investigation of the primary stability agree with the abovementioned ex vivo studies. Using the RFA, the author found statistically significant differences in the primary stability measurements of the iliac crest flap and the fibula flap. Statistical differences were found between the measurement immediately after implant placement, but not after implant healing (osseointegration).

In contrast, for the secondary stability, no differences are reported between the fibula and the iliac crest flap. The comparison between primary and secondary stability proved a significant decrease of the implant-bone interface stability for the fibula and a significant increase in the iliac crest. This phenomenon is known from other issues.

The author concluded that the bone remodeling during the osseointegration process after dental implant placement in free revascularized bone flaps is independent of the initial bone density and would be similar after the implant healing period between fibula and iliac crest flap [15].

References

1. Urken ML, Weinberg H, Vickery C, Buchbinder D, Lawson W, Biller HF. Oromandibular reconstruction using microvascular composite free flaps. Report of 71 cases and a new classification scheme for bony, soft-tissue, and neurologic defects. Arch Otolaryngol Head Neck Surg. 1991;117(7):733–44.
2. Sjöström M, Sennerby L, Nilson H, Lundgren S. Reconstruction of the atrophic edentulous maxilla with free iliac crest grafts and implants: a 3-year report of a prospective clinical study. Clin Implant Dent Relat Res. 2007;9:46–59.
3. Esposito M, Hirsch JM, Lekholm U, Thomsen P. Biological factors contributing to failures of osseointegrated oral implants. (I). Successcriteria and epidemiology. Eur J Oral Sci. 1998;106:527–51.

4. Sennerby L, Meredith N. Implant stability measurements using resonance frequency analysis: biological and biomechanical aspects and clinical implications. Periodontol 2000. 2008;47:51–66.
5. Bertossi D, Bissolotti G, Corrocher G, Anesi A, Nocini P-F. O.301 The use of tapered dental implants in severe jaw atrophies. J Craniomaxillofac Surg. 2008;36:S76. https://doi.org/10.1016/S1010-5182(08)71425-2.
6. Atieh MA, Alsabeeha NHM, Tawse-Smith A, Duncan WJ. Piezoelectric versus conventional implant site preparation: a systematic review and metaanalysis. Clin Implant Dent Relat Res. 2018;20:261–70.
7. Anesi A, Ferretti M, Cavani F, Salvatori R, Bianchi M, Russo A, Chiarini L, Palumbo C. Structural and ultrastructural analyses of bone regeneration in rabbit cranial osteotomy: Piezosurgery versus traditional osteotomes. J Craniomaxillofac Surg. 2018;46(1):107–18. https://doi.org/10.1016/j.jcms.2017.10.004. Epub 2017 Oct 12.
8. Bardyn T, Gédet P, Hallermann W, Büchler P. Quantifying the influence of bone density and thickness on resonance frequency analysis: an in vitro study of biomechanical test materials. Int J Oral Maxillofac Implants. 2009;24:1006–14.
9. Meredith N, Alleyne D, Cawley P. Quantitative determination of the stability of the implant-tissue interface using resonance frequency analysis. Clin Oral Implants Res. 1996;7:261–7.
10. Trisi P, Perfetti G, Baldoni E, Berardi D, Colagiovanni M, Scogna G. Implant micromotion is related to peak insertion torque and bone density. Clin Oral Implants Res. 2009;20:467–71.
11. Pagliani L, Sennerby L, Petersson A, Verrocchi D, Volpe S, Andersson P. The relationship between resonance frequency analysis (RFA) and lateral displacement of dental implants: an in vitro study. J Oral Rehabil. 2013;40:221–7.
12. Sim CP, Lang NP. Factors influencing resonance frequency analysis assessed by Osstell mentor during implant tissue integration: I. Instrument positioning, bone structure, implant length. Clin Oral Implants Res. 2010;21:598–604.
13. Kahraman S, Bal BT, Asar NV, Turkyilmaz I, Tözüm TF. Clinical study on the insertion torque and wireless resonance frequency analysis in the assessment of torque capacity and stability of self-tapping dental implants. J Oral Rehabil. 2009;36:755–61.
14. Song YD, Jun SH, Kwon JJ. Correlation between bone quality evaluated by cone-beam computerized tomography and implant primary stability. Int J Oral Maxillofac Implants. 2009;24:59–64.
15. Möhlhenrich SC, Kniha K, Elvers D, Ayoub N, Goloborodko E, Hölzle F, et al. Intraosseous stability of dental implants in free revascularized fibula and iliac crest bone flaps. J Craniomaxillofac Surg. 2016;44(12):1935–9.
16. Mertens C, Decker C, Engel M, Sander A, Hoffmann J, Freier K. Early bone resorption of free microvascular reanastomized bone grafts for mandibular reconstruction–a comparison of iliac crest and fibula grafts. J Craniomaxillofac Surg. 2014;42(5):e217–23.
17. Akkocaoglu M, Cehreli MC, Tekdemir I, Comert A, Güzel E, Dağdeviren A, et al. Primary stability of simultaneously placed dental implants in extraoral donor graft sites: a human cadaver study. J Oral Maxillofac Surg. 2007;65(3):400–7.

Part VI

Adjunct Procedures

Second Vascularized Fibula Flap and Osteotomy to Correct Malocclusion

Pier Francesco Nocini, Alexandre Anesi, and Luigi Chiarini

Second Vascularized Fibula Flap

For alveolar bone augmentation, a further reconstructive procedure is possible with a new revascularized fibula flap fixed onto the surface of the first fibula, placed as reconstruction of the basal bone of the mandible.

A good patient-surgeon relationship is needed, because a further major surgical intervention is proposed to restore the natural height of the mandibular symphysis and to allow for dental rehabilitation.

Two consecutive vascularized free flaps are reported in a small series of patients affected by recurrent squamous cell carcinoma. The two flaps have reconstructed the mandible from angle-to-angle. The need for rapid and uncomplicated bone healing of compromised tissues after radiation therapy justifies this reconstructive option. The bone union between the two flaps was good, and it supported the planning for dental implant placement to restore the masticatory function. The authors reported that donor site morbidity was negligible [1–3].

We have demonstrated that the mandible reconstruction with the fibula flap is feasible and does not influence the natural course of the primary disease in BRONJ-resected patients [4].

Two consecutive vascularized free flaps constitute a valid reconstructive option to achieve rapid healing after salvage surgery for recurrent oral cancer [3].

Furthermore, a second fibula vascularized flap is reliable for simultaneous augmentation in symphysis, parasymphysis, and the premolar area over a previous fibula flap: implant-borne dental rehabilitation becomes practicable to improve quality of speech and diet. Large mandibular defects due to BRONJ, osteonecrosis, or major trauma may be fully restored with acceptable donor site morbidity (Figs. 1–3) [5].

The unoperated side of the neck is the first choice for preparing the recipient vessels [3]. We demonstrated that osteotomies performed using piezosurgical devices show more advanced stages of bone healing compared with rotary instruments. Moreover, even more powerful devices (output power of 75 W) do not alter the process of bone healing. Generally speaking, we recommend piezosurgical devices for improved bone healing when osteotomies are planned in all primary and secondary phases of the reconstruction with a fibula flap [6–9].

Secondary Osteotomies to Correct Malocclusion

Malocclusion and asymmetric facial contour may follow reconstruction of the jaws with vascularized fibula flap for an inaccurate insetting procedure. The misaligned reconstructed jaw may influence the implant placement, resulting in occlusal overload that may impair the long-term survival of implant-supported prostheses [10]. Correction of malocclusion after fibula graft may be obtained by secondary osteotomies [11].

We described the use of a Le Fort osteotomy to correct malocclusion after fibula flap reconstruction of the maxilla (Figs. 4–9) [12].

Six months after fibula transfer, and with complete healing, maxillo-mandibular relationships and centric occlusion have to be recorded to plan secondary osteotomies. Preoperative planning to finalization of occlusion can be prepared by examination of dental models in an occlusal articulator, of face bow, and diagnostic wax-up, to define the occlusal vertical dimension and the proper dental volume. Clinical photographs were taken at the preoperative stage.

P. F. Nocini (✉)
Division of Oral and Maxillo-Facial Surgery, University Hospital of Verona, Verona, Italy
e-mail: pierfrancesco.nocini@univr.it

A. Anesi · L. Chiarini
Cranio-Maxillo-Facial Surgery Unit, University Hospital of Modena, Modena, Italy
e-mail: alexandre.anesi@unimore.it; luigi.chiarini@unimore.it

G. De Santis et al. (eds.), *Atlas of Mandibular and Maxillary Reconstruction with the Fibula Flap*,
https://doi.org/10.1007/978-3-030-10684-3_13

Preoperative lateral and panoramic radiographs and non-contrast maxillofacial computed tomography (CT) scan with 1 mm cuts are scheduled. If the patient lacks adequate dental space and is not suitable for implant-supported prosthetic restoration, a corrective mandibular osteotomy or a Le Fort I osteotomy can be planned to restore the occlusal relationships between the jaws. The operative fundamentals for improving hard and soft tissue contours are not dissimilar from those for orthognathic surgery. It is also possible to transform the diagnostic wax-up into an acrylic splint to assist bone repositioning during surgery. We demonstrated that osteotomies performed using piezosurgergical devices show more advanced stages of bone healing compared with rotary instruments. Moreover, even more powerful devices (output power of 75W) do not alter the process of bone healing. Generally speaking, we recommend piezosurgical devices for improved bone healing when osteotomies are planned [6].

The intervention for malocclusion correction after fibula reconstruction allows the direct assessment of complete bone union between the fibula and the native bone, along with the simultaneous removal of the plates and screws. The ideal dental relationships of the osteotomized and moved jaw can be established by using a surgical acrylic splint, which is secured to the opposing dentition. The peroneal vessels can be ligated on this occasion, enabling the osteotomized jaw to

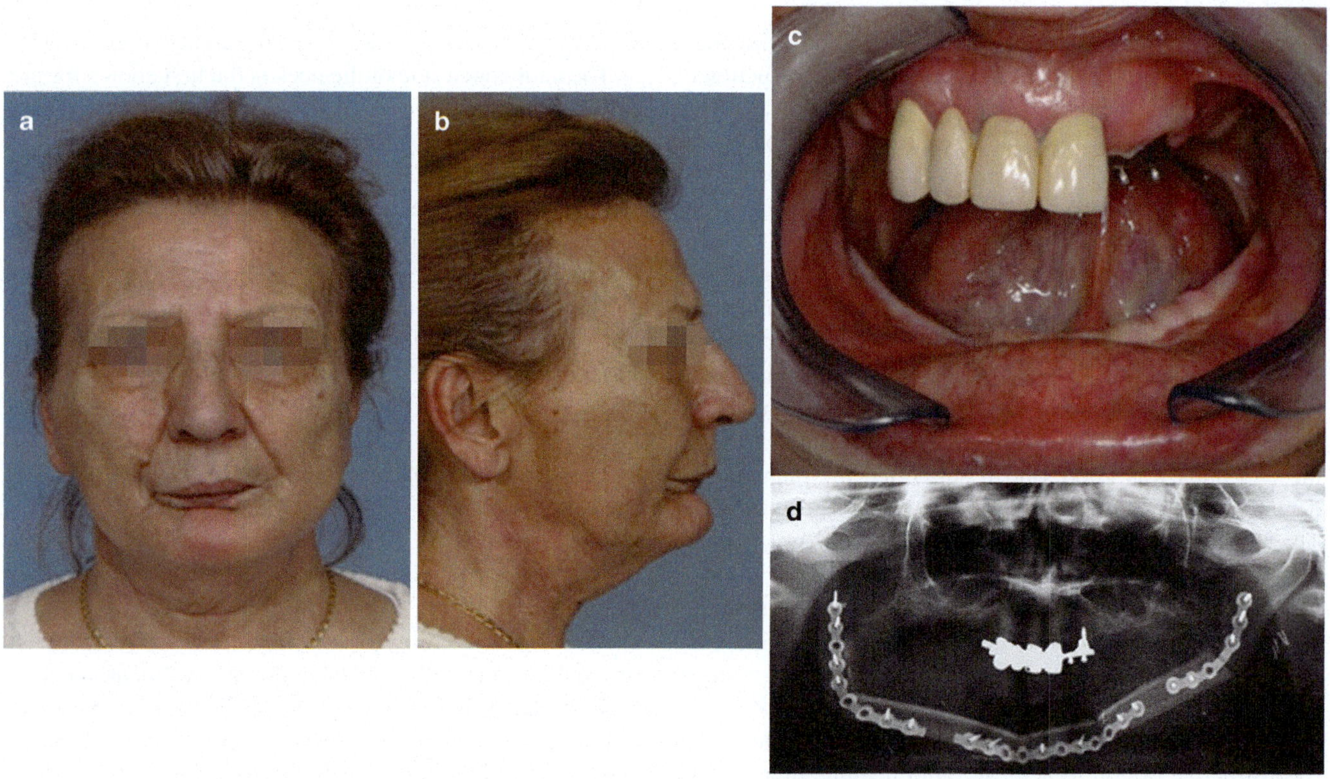

Fig. 1 The patient previously underwent subtotal mandibulectomy for bisphosphonate-related osteonecrosis of the jaw (BRONJ) associated with intravenous infusion of zoledronic acid; fibula free flap reconstruction was previously carried out. (**a** and **b**) Remaining facial asymmetry and malocclusion were present. (**c** and **d**) Mandibular vertical bone discrepancy was evident. No implant-borne prosthetic rehabilitation could be planned

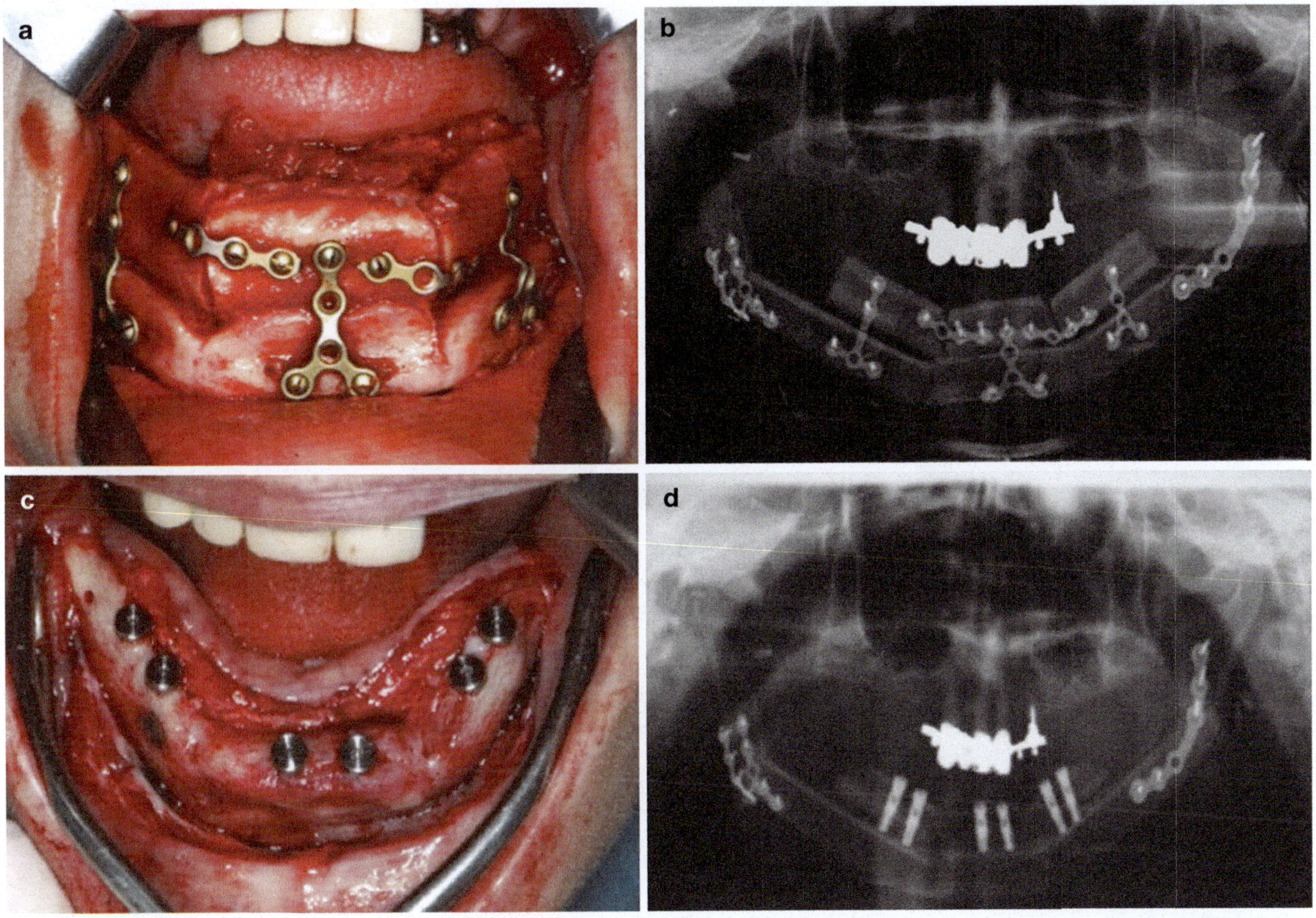

Fig. 2 (**a** and **b**) Corrective osteotomies were performed along with mandibular height increase through a second fibular flap. (**c**) Endosseous dental implant were correctly placed in restored alveolar bone. (**d**) Postoperative orthopantomograph

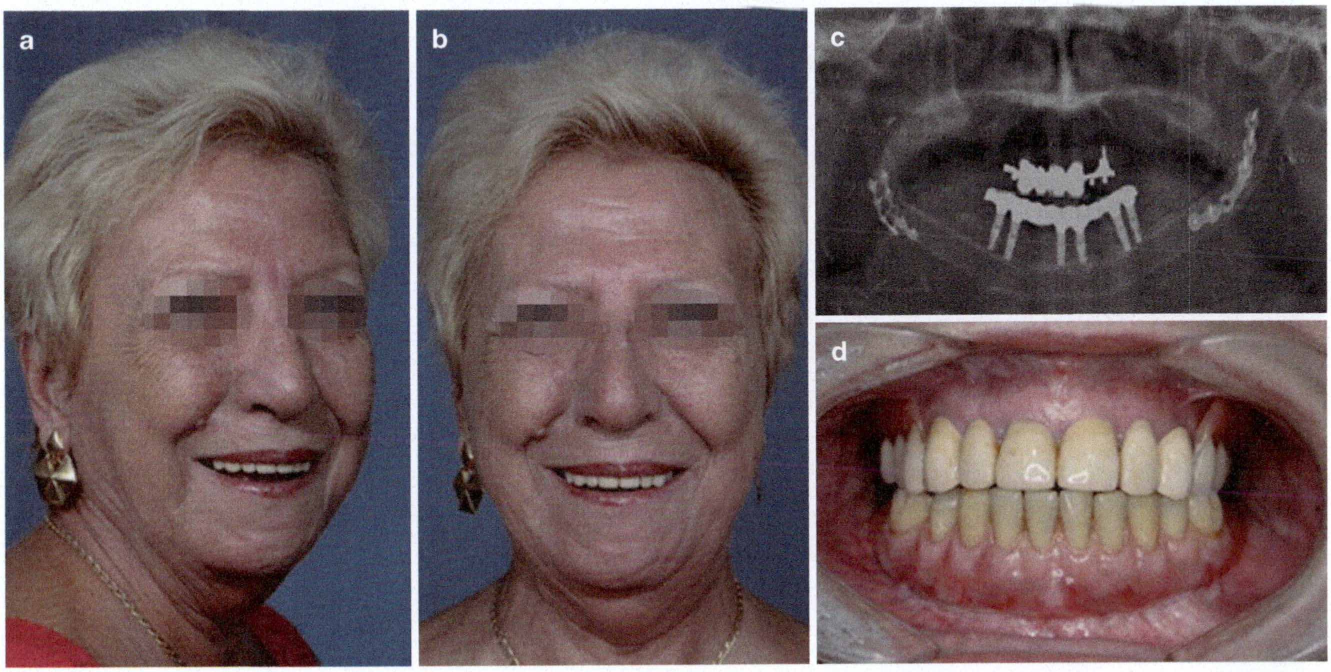

Fig. 3 (**a** and **b**) Final result with implant-borne prosthetic rehabilitation, stable after 5 years. (**c**) Final panoramic radiograph with implant-borne prosthetic rehabilitation. (**d**) The final dental status with implant-borne prosthetic rehabilitation

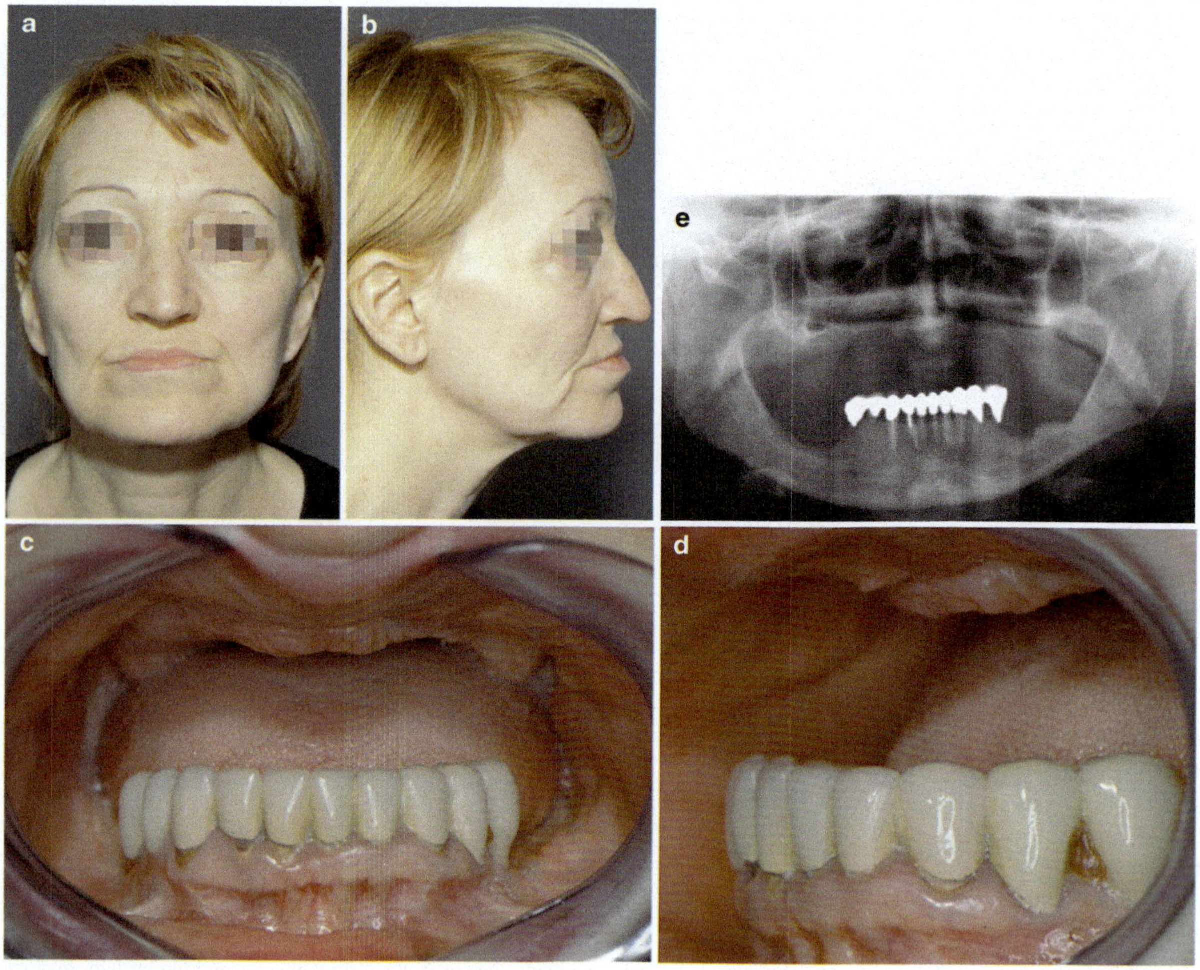

Fig. 4 (**a** and **b**) Preoperative frontal and lateral views of the patient. (**c** and **d**) Inadequate prosthetic space related to extreme upper jaw bone atrophy. (**e**) Extreme maxillary atrophy also was evident in orthopantomograph

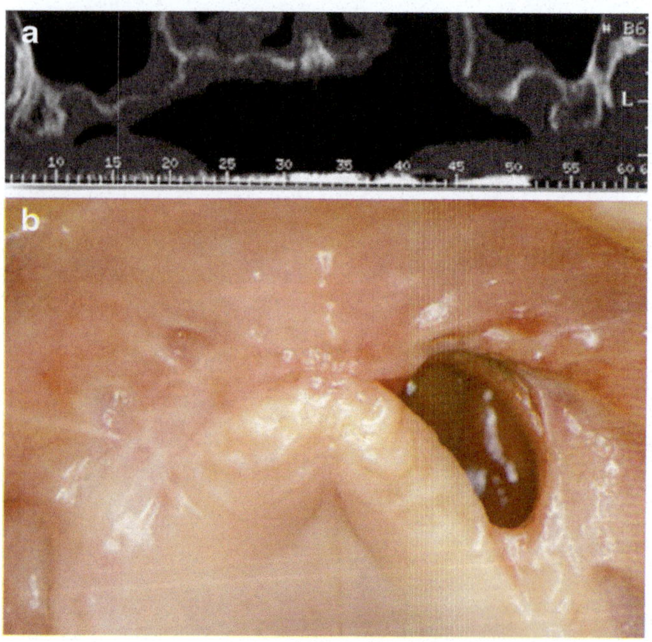

Fig. 5 (**a** and **b**) Extreme maxillary atrophy is associated to a large oro-antral fistula, detectable both on CT coronal reconstruction and in oral examination

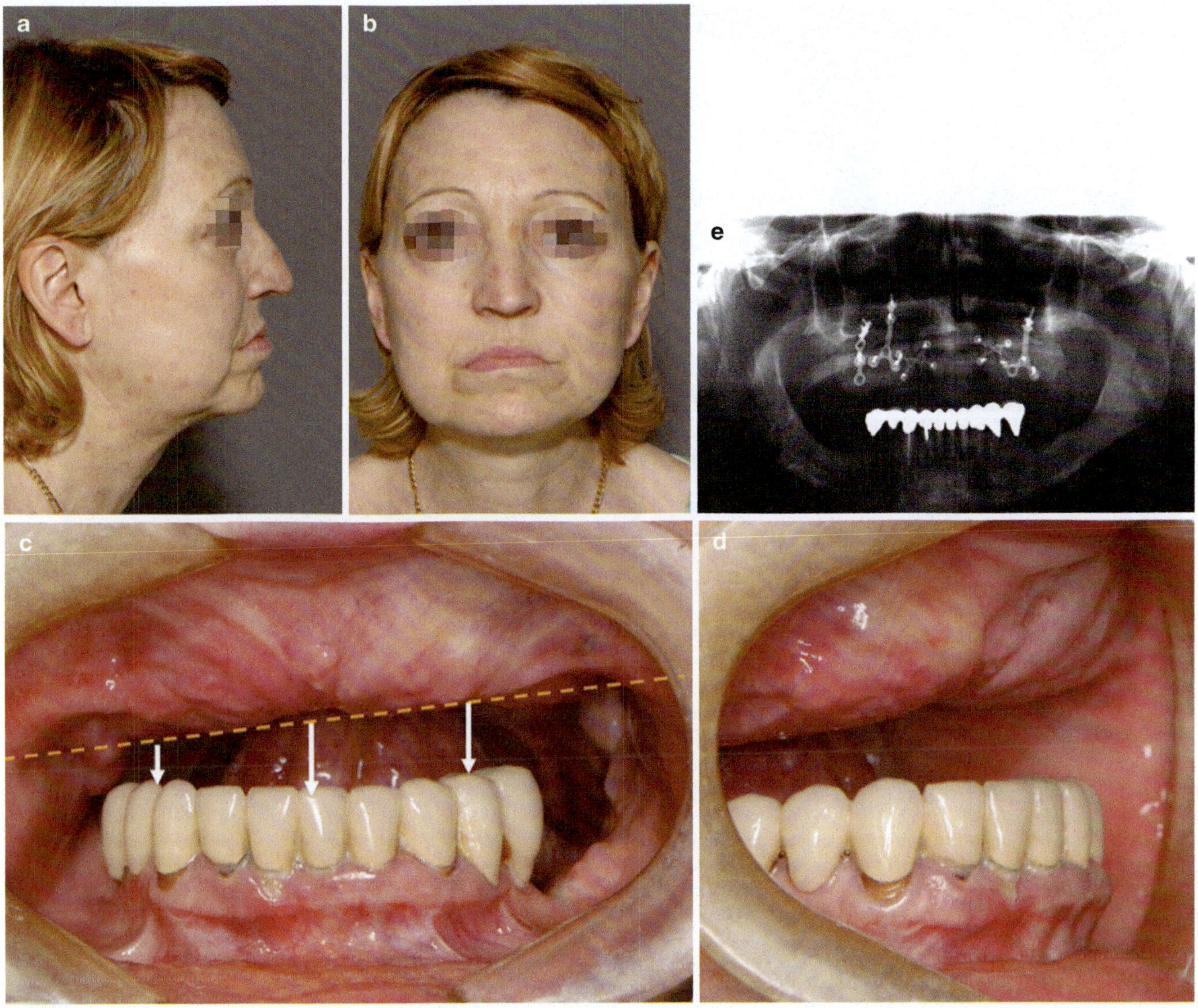

Fig. 6 (**a** and **b**) Patient's appearance 3 months after fibula free flap reconstruction. (**c** and **d**) Intraoral view showing the lack of prosthetic space owing to canting of the fibula on the right side. (**e**) Orthopantomograph showed advanced bone healing process of the fibula

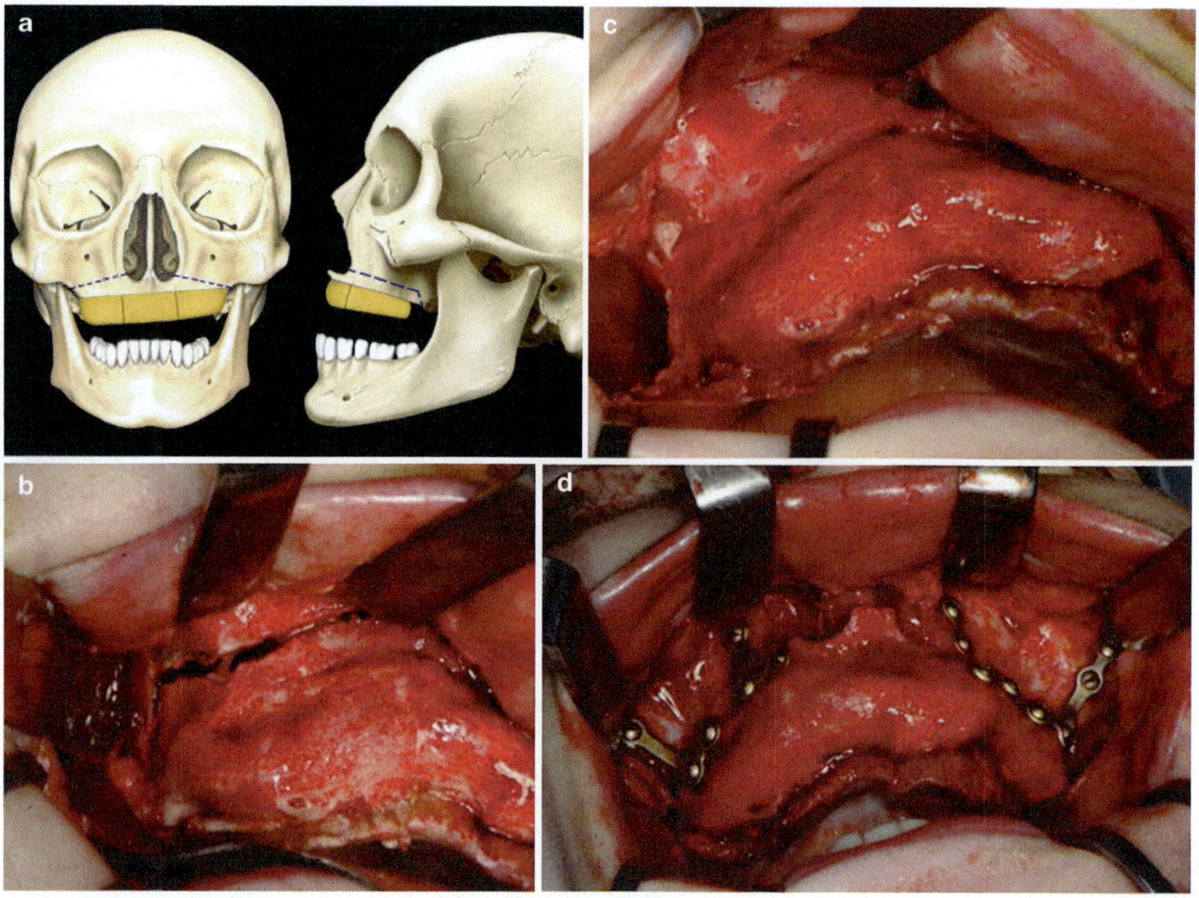

Fig. 7 (**a**) Drawing for osteotomic lines planning necessary to move the maxilla forward and downward. (**b**) Intraoperative bone marking for Le Fort I osteotomy. (**c**) Le Fort I osteotomy: intraoperative view. (**d**) Intraoperative view of complete bone union between fibula and basal bone of maxilla 6 months after fibula reconstruction

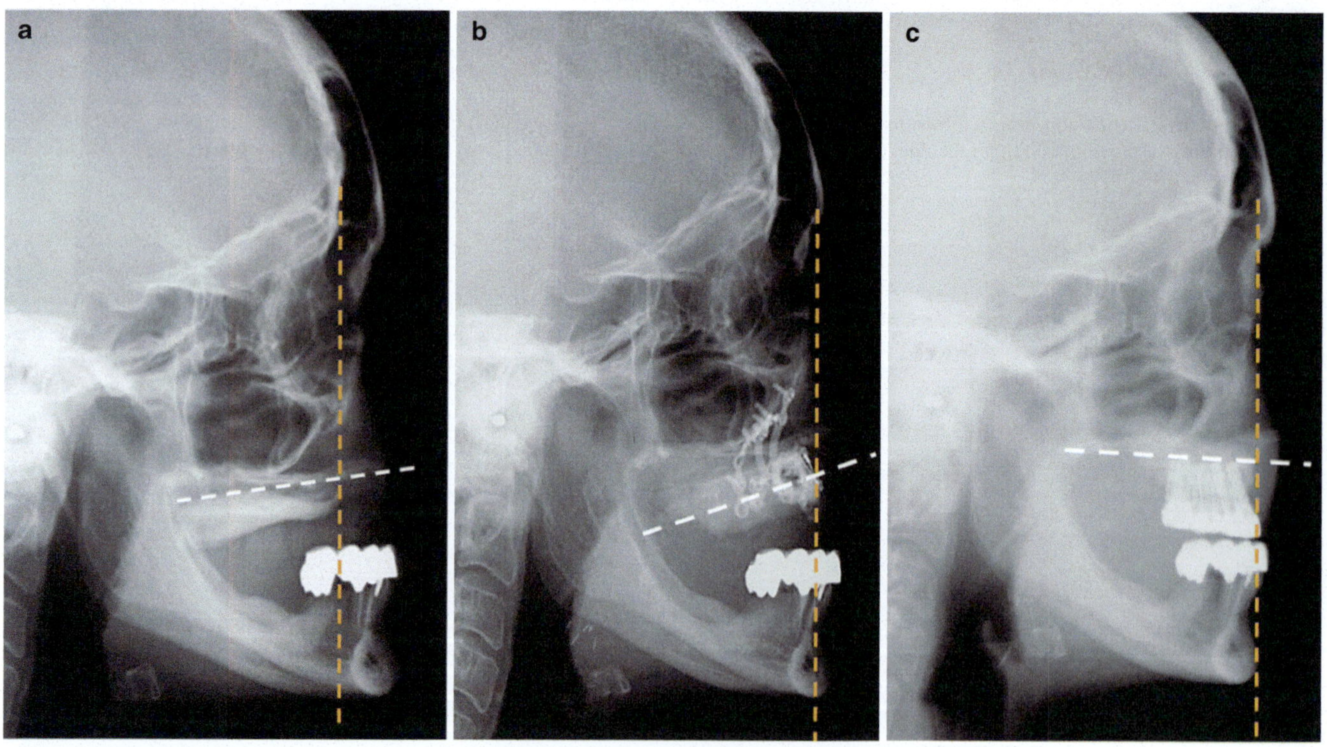

Fig. 8 Comparison between lateral teleradiographs during the course of correction of the malocclusion. (**a**) Initial maxillary atrophic plane. (**b**) After fibula flap transfer. (**c**) Final positioned maxillary plane, after corrective Le Fort I osteotomy

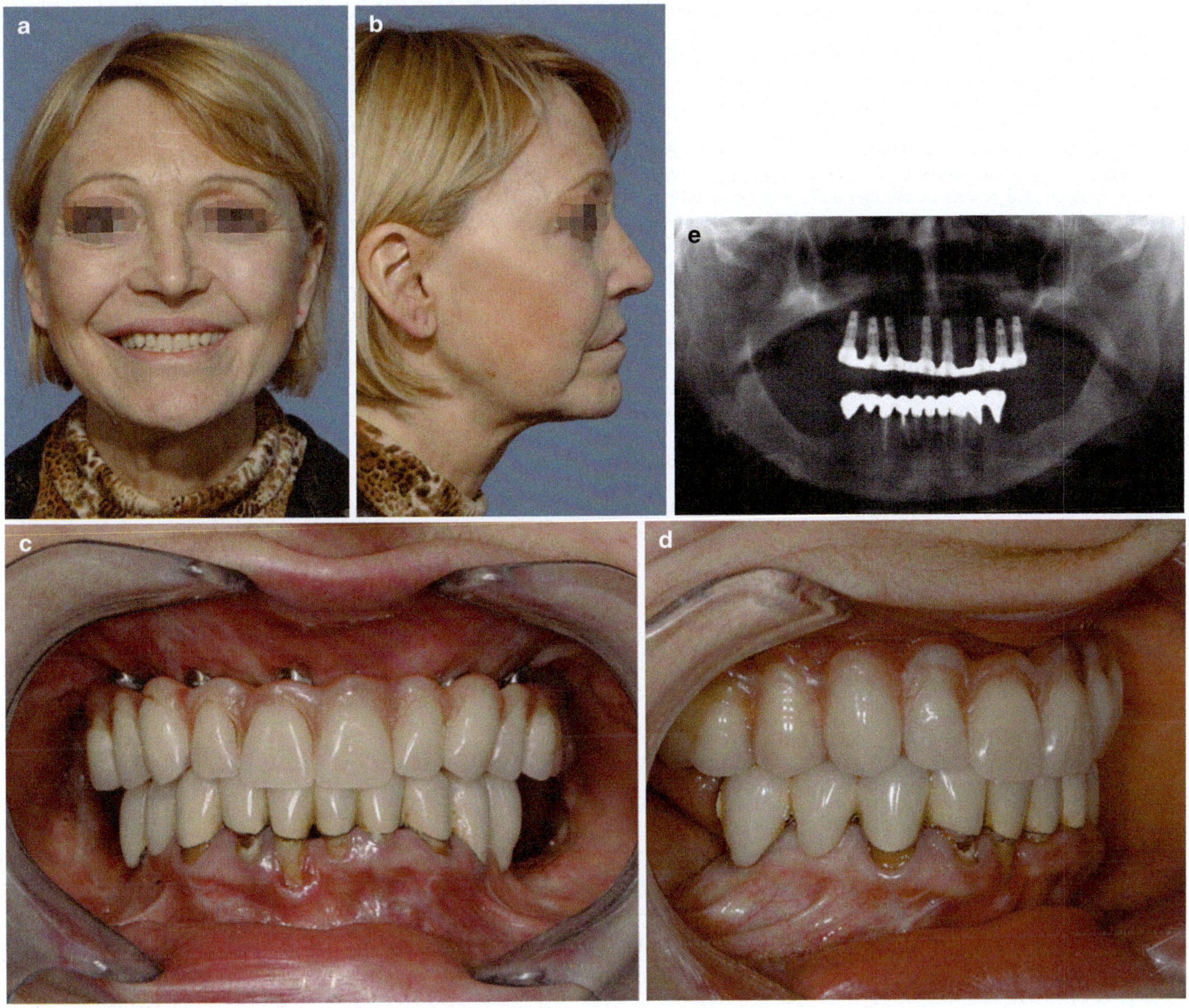

Fig. 9 (**a** and **b**) Postoperative frontal and lateral views of the patient. (**c** and **d**) Final implant-borne prosthetic rehabilitation. (**e**) Orthopantomograph at completion of dental implant-borne prosthetic rehabilitation

move with more ease and thus proceed according to the planning. The correct jaw position needs rigid fixation with 2.0 screws and miniplates. A further intervention for removal of plates and screws is required 3 months later; endosseous dental implants can be placed at once [13].

Nowadays virtual computer planning promotes a more accurate analysis of dentofacial deformity. A three-dimensional (3D) reconstruction of a preoperative non-contrast maxillofacial computed tomography (CT) scan with 1 mm cuts or a cone beam CT may be planned. Virtual surgical planning uses specific software that elaborates CT data: the mid-facial osteotomy or mandibular osteotomy is simulated. According with the virtual surgical planning, a custom titanium plate can be prepared for rapid and accurate orientation of the occlusal plane.

References

1. Jones NF, Elahi MM. Osteosynthesis and bony healing between two consecutive free fibular bone grafts. Plast Reconstr Surg. 2000;105(1):166–70.
2. Lutz BS, Bagenholm T, Adell R. Angle-to-angle mandibular reconstruction with two free fibular flaps in a patient with two consecutive gingival cancers. Scand J Plast Reconstr Surg Hand Surg. 2004;38:46–9.
3. Matros E, Schwarz GS, Mehrara BJ, Hu QY, Cordeiro PG, Disa JJ. Indications and outcomes for mandibular reconstruc-

tion using sequential bilateral fibula flaps. Plast Reconstr Surg. 2010;126(5):1539–47.
4. Nocini PF, Saia G, Bettini G, Ragazzo M, Blandamura S, Chiarini L, et al. Vascularized fibula flap reconstruction of the mandible in bisphosphonate-related osteonecrosis. Eur J Surg Oncol. 2009;35(4):373–9.
5. Bedogni A, Anesi A, Fior A, Bettini G, Nocini PF. Microsurgical reconstruction of the mandible in a patient with evans syndrome: a case report and review of the literature. J Reconstr Microsurg. 2013;29(8):545–50.
6. Anesi A, Ferretti M, Cavani F, Salvatori R, Bianchi M, Russo A, Chiarini L, Palumbo C. Structural and ultrastructural analyses of bone regeneration in rabbit cranial osteotomy: piezosurgery versus traditional osteotomes. J Craniomaxillofac Surg. 2018;46(1):107–18. https://doi.org/10.1016/j.jcms.2017.10.004. Epub 2017 Oct 12.
7. Turra M, Bertossi D, Bissolotti G, Anesi A, Chiarini L, Nocini PF. O.095 Genioplasty with piezosurgery. J Craniomaxillofac Surg. 2008;36(Suppl1):S24. https://doi.org/10.1016/S1010-5182(08)71219-8.
8. Nocini PF, Turra M, Valsecchi S, Blandamura S, Bedogni A. Microvascular free bone flap harvest with piezosurgery. J Oral Maxillofac Surg. 2011;69(5):1485–92. https://doi.org/10.1016/j.joms.2009.10.016. Epub 2010 Jun 29.
9. Chiarini L, Albanese M, Anesi A, Galzignato PF, Mortellaro C, Nocini P, Bertossi D. Surgical treatment of unilateral condylar hyperplasia with piezosurgery. J Craniofac Surg. 2014;25(3):808–10. https://doi.org/10.1097/SCS.0000000000000699.
10. Bertossi D, Bissolotti G, Corrocher G, Anesi A, Nocini PF. O.301 The use of tapered dental implants in severe jaw atrophies. J Craniomaxillofac Surg. 2008;36(Suppl1):S76. https://doi.org/10.1016/S1010-5182(08)71425-2.
11. Kim Y, Oh TJ, Misch CE, Wang HL. Occlusal considerations in implant therapy: clinical guidelines with biomechanical rationale. Clin Oral Implants Res. 2005;16(1):26–35.
12. Nocini PF, Chiarini L, Fior A, Bedogni A. Le Fort I osteotomy to correct malocclusion after reconstruction of the maxilla with the free fibula flap. J Craniofac Surg. 2009;20(5):1420–3.
13. Nocini PF, De Santis G, Bedogni A, Chiarini L. Simultaneous bimaxillary alveolar ridge augmentation by a single free fibular transfer: a case report. J Craniomaxillofac Surg. 2002;30:46–53.

Secondary Procedures and Refinements

Alessio Baccarani, Marta Starnoni, and Giorgio De Santis

The jaw cosmetically defines the lower third of the face and is essential for normal mastication, swallowing, and speech.

To achieve both functionally and cosmetically favorable results, it is advisable to avoid vertical discrepancy between the grafted fibula and the residual maxillary stumps [1]. A number of technical options may be used to overcome this. Double-barreling the fibula increases its height for accepting osteointegrated dental implants [2–4]. Alternatively, vertical distraction osteogenesis can increase the height of a single-strut fibula, but the process alters internal bony architecture [5–7]. Finally, a second-stage bone graft over the fibula can be inset [8–10], if adequate soft tissue coverage is warranted.

Whenever feasible, double-barreling the fibula is the option of choice for several reasons, including outcomes of immediate height increase, no need for further surgical procedures, and earlier functional rehabilitation with osteointegrated dental implants [11].

The highly vascularized fibula flap has the capacity to revascularize adjacent bone or cartilaginous graft if these are required as an accessory specimen in the reconstruction. The vascularized periosteum of the fibula flap has been demonstrated to quickly and easily integrate into the surrounding tissues; thus, arterial ligation after 10 days does not compromise flap viability. Standard X-ray, magnetic resonance imaging, bone scintigraphy, and SPECT can be used to detect the revascularization of the adjacent graft. This method can be applied successfully when the temporomandibular joint condyle needs to be reconstructed [12, 13]. The metatarsal head can be used as a bone graft. The same principle of revascularization of adjacent tissues can be used when vertical mandible height must be restored. In this case, an alternative to the double-barrel or other more recent techniques is the use of iliac bone graft inset on the fibula flap to augment the mandibular ridge [14].

Despite the possibility of inserting implants into the fibula during primary reconstruction [4, 15–17], we advocate a delayed implant rehabilitation to avoid potential implant loss upon flap failure, complex preoperative planning, implant malpositioning, mucosal lesions, and implant exposure during adjuvant radiotherapy, given the often-unpredictable course of the disease being treated [18]. In this perspective, we usually plan implant insertion about 6 months after surgery.

Furthermore, even if at present, limited evidence exists regarding the number of implants that are required to adequately support fixed dentures in patients with reconstructed jaws, our experience suggests that a single implant per tooth is the best option. The advantages include superior durability of the prosthesis and a superior masticatory strength.

The use of vascularized bone grafts and placement of endosteal implants are intended to help restore function and aesthetics following mandibular resection. However, excessive thickness and mobility of the overlying skin and soft tissue and obliteration of the vestibule limit the use of endosteal implants for oral rehabilitation [19]. Implants surrounded by mobile soft tissue may promote inflammatory changes and pocket formation [20–23]. On the other hand, the keratinized tissue surrounding implant abutments tends to be less subject to peri-implant inflammation [24, 25].

We suggest procedures to eliminate compromised peri-implant soft tissue and to attempt to recreate the properties of native gingiva with the mucosa rigidly adhering to the neomandible. These procedures include tissue thinning during grafting, excision of redundant soft tissue, split-thickness skin graft, palatal mucosal grafts, and vestibuloplasty.

A. Baccarani · M. Starnoni · G. De Santis (✉)
Plastic and Reconstructive Surgery Unit, University Hospital of Modena, Modena, Italy
e-mail: alessio.baccarani@unimore.it; giorgio.desantis@unimore.it

G. De Santis et al. (eds.), *Atlas of Mandibular and Maxillary Reconstruction with the Fibula Flap*,
https://doi.org/10.1007/978-3-030-10684-3_14

If soft tissue management is inadequate, risks can be poor hygiene around implants, hyperplastic peri-implant tissue, and soft tissue infections with eventual implant loss [26, 27].

Finally, but equally important, significant aesthetic improvement is offered by autologous fat transfer that allows for the correction of contour deformities, restoration of the volume, improvement of the scar quality, and treatment of contracted scars. Scar revision as well as all the minor surgical procedures in the plastic surgeons' armamentarium (such as laser therapy, local flaps, Z-plasty) provide our reconstructed patients with the possibility of further superior cosmetic results (Figs. 1–10).

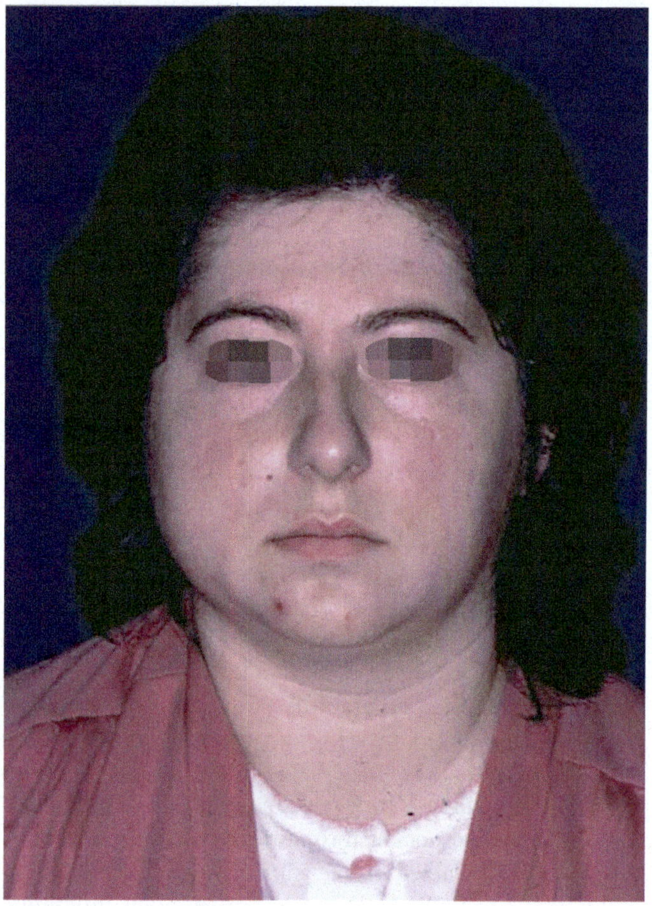

Fig. 1 Case 1: Preoperative view of a patient affected by ameloblastoma odontogenic cyst of the right mandibular angle

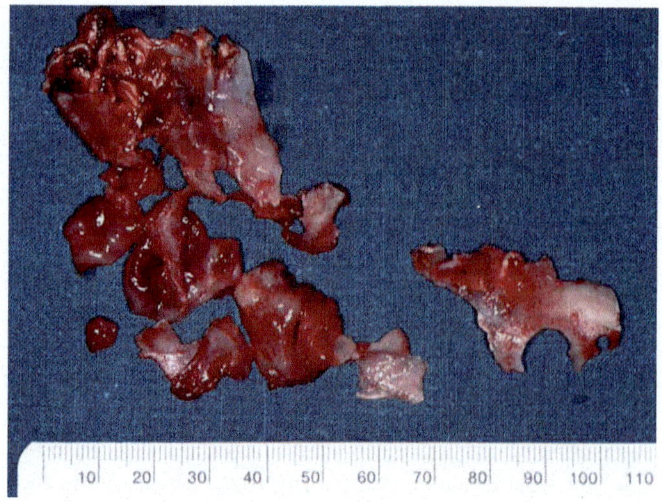

Fig. 2 Case 1: Resected specimen

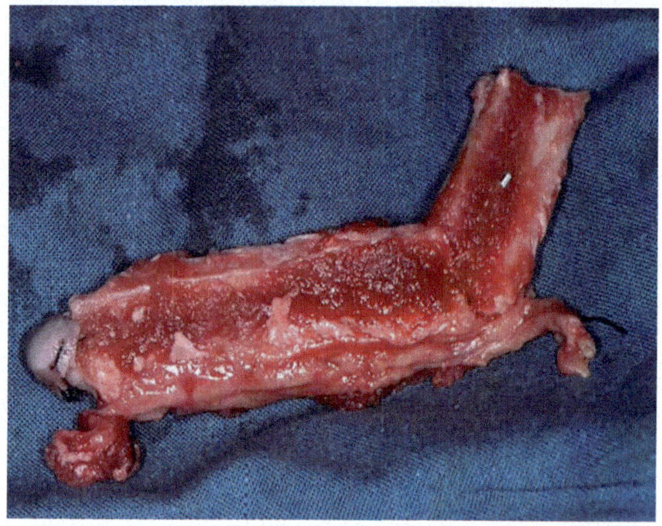

Fig. 3 Case 1: Two-segment harvested fibular flap including metatarsal head for condyle reconstruction

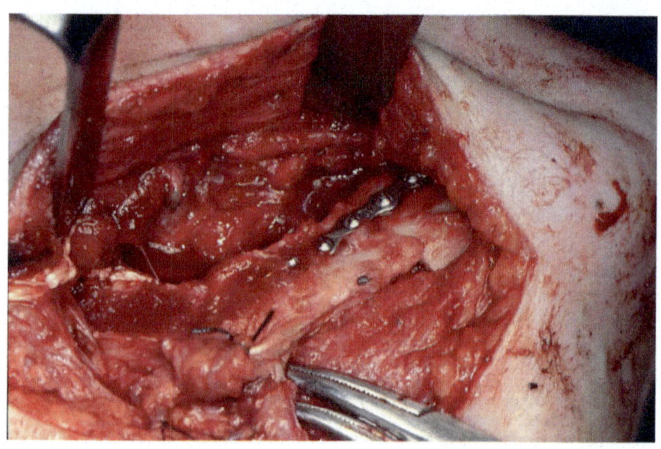

Fig. 4 Case 1: Flap inset after revascularization

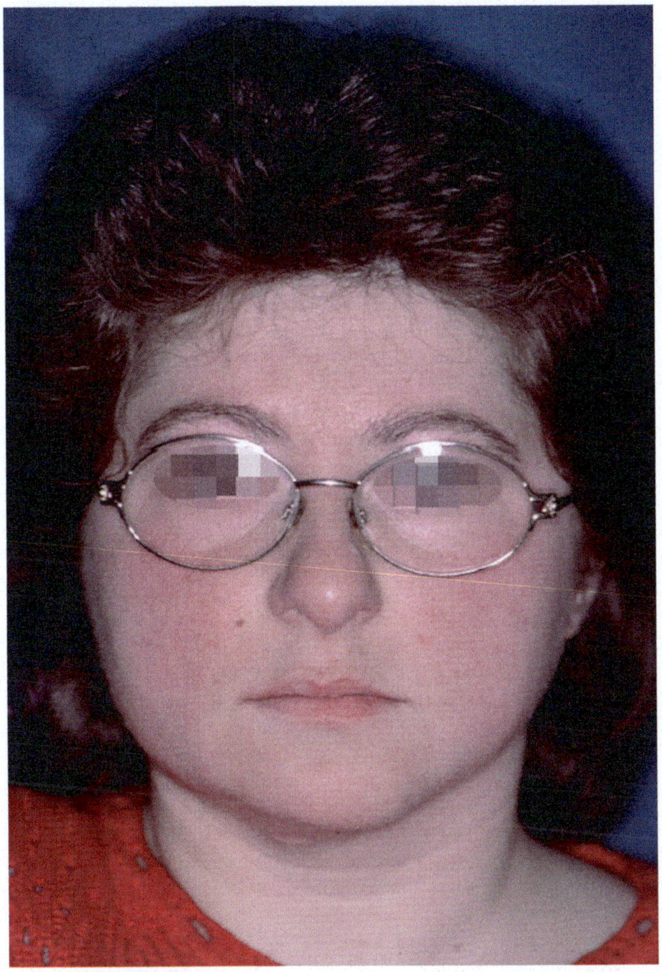

Fig. 5 Case 1: One-year postoperative view

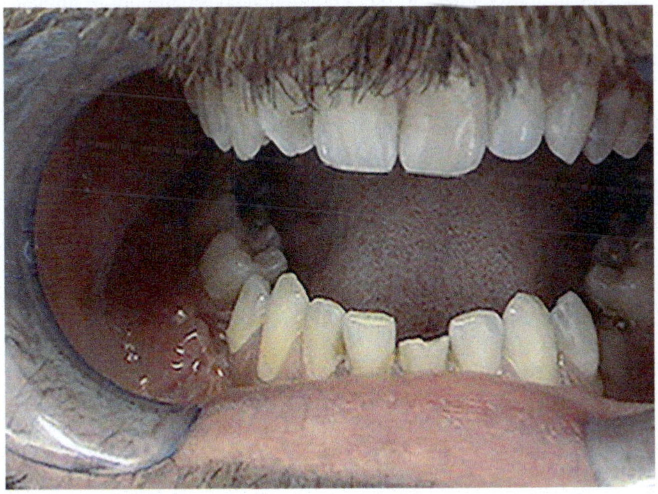

Fig. 6 Case 2: Intraoral view of a patient affected by ameloblastoma of the mandible [26, 27]

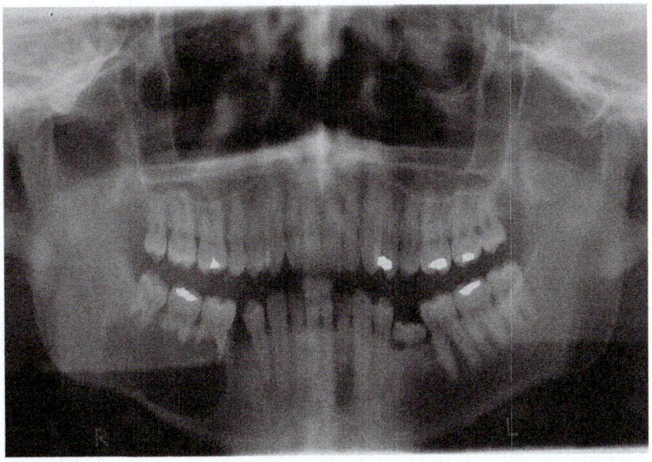

Fig. 7 Case 2: Radiogram of the lesion involving the right hemi-mandible

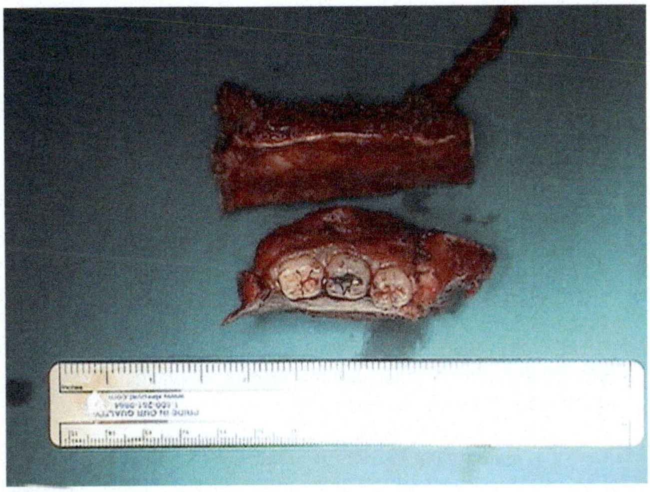

Fig. 8 Case 2: Resected specimen and harvested single-strut fibula flap

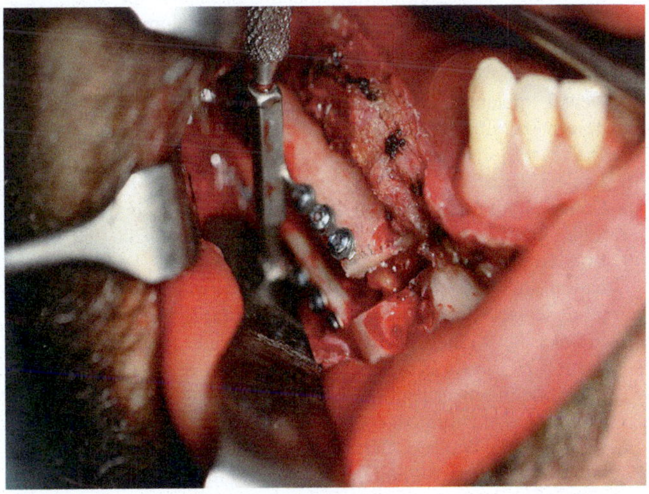

Fig. 9 Case 2: Vertical discrepancy was managed by distraction osteogenesis

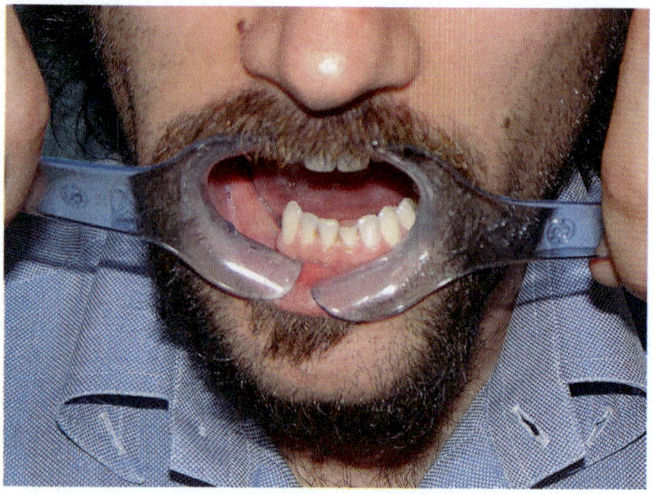

Fig. 10 Case 2: One-year post-op after secondary procedure

References

1. Yim KK, Wei FQ. Fibula osteoseptocutaneous flap for mandible reconstruction. Microsurgery. 1994;15:245, 19949.
2. Wallace CG, Chang YM, Tsai CY, Wei FC. Harnessing the potential of the free fibula osteoseptocutaneous flap in mandible reconstruction. Plast Reconstr Surg. 2010;125:305–14.
3. Chang YM, Tsai CY, Wei FC. One-stage, double-barrel fibula osteoseptocutaneous flap and immediate dental implants for functional and aesthetic reconstruction of segmental mandibular defects. Plast Reconstr Surg. 2008;122:143–5.
4. Chang YM, Wallace CG, Tsai CY, Shen YF, Hsu YM, Wei FC. Dental implant outcome after primary implantation into double-barreled fibula osteoseptocutaneous free flap-reconstructed mandible. Plast Reconstr Surg. 2011;128:1220–8.
5. Iizuka T, Hallermann W, Seto I, Smolka W, Smolka K, Bosshardt DD. Bi-directional distraction osteogenesis of the alveolar bone using an extraosseous device. Clin Oral Implants Res. 2005;16:700–7.
6. Klesper B, Lazar F, Siessegger M, Hidding J, Zöller JE. Vertical distraction osteogenesis of fibula transplants for mandibular reconstruction: a preliminary study. J Craniomaxillofac Surg. 2002;30:280–5.
7. Chenping Z, Min R, Liqun X, Yongjie H, Wenjun Y, Tong J, et al. Dental implant distractor combined with free fibular flap: a new design for simultaneous functional mandibular reconstruction. J Oral Maxillofac Surg. 2012;70(11):2687–700.
8. Lee JH, Kim MJ, Choi WS, Yoon PY, Ahn KM, Myung H, et al. Concomitant reconstruction of mandibular basal and alveolar bone with a free fibular flap. Int J Oral Maxillofac Surg. 2004;33:150–6.
9. Li L, Blake F, Heiland M, Schmelzle R, Pohlenz P. Longterm evaluation after mandibular reconstruction with fibular grafts versus microsurgical fibular flaps. J Oral Maxillofac Surg. 2007;65:281–6.
10. Smolka K, Kraehenbuehl M, Eggensperger N, Hallermann W, Thoren H, Iizuka T, et al. Fibula free flap reconstruction of the mandible in cancer patients: evaluation of a combined surgical and prosthodontic treatment concept. Oral Oncol. 2008;44:571–81.
11. Chang YM, Wallace CG, Hsu YM, Shen YF, Tsai CY, Wei FC. Outcome of osseointegrated dental implants in double-barrel and vertically distracted fibula osteoseptocutaneous free flaps for segmental mandibular defect reconstruction. Plast Reconstr Surg. 2014;134:1033–43.
12. Anesi A, Ferretti M, Cavani F, Salvatori R, Bianchi M, Russo A, Chiarini L, Palumbo C. Structural and ultrastructural analyses of bone regeneration in rabbit cranial osteotomy: Piezosurgery versus traditional osteotomes. J Craniomaxillofac Surg. 2018;46(1):107–18. https://doi.org/10.1016/j.jcms.2017.10.004. Epub 2017 Oct 12.
13. Chiarini L, Albanese M, Anesi A, Galzignato PF, Mortellaro C, Nocini PF, Bertossi D. Surgical Treatment of Unilateral Condylar Hyperplasia With Piezosurgery. J Craniofac Surg. 2014;25(3):808–10.
14. De Santis G, Pinelli M, Gargano F, Baccarani A. Aesthetic and functional innovations in jaw reconstruction with free fibula flap. In: Eisenmann-Klein M, Neuhann-Lorenz C, editors. Innovations in plastic and aesthetic surgery. Berlin: Springer; 2008.
15. Roumanas ED, Markowitz BL, Lorant JA, Calcaterra TC, Jones NF, Beumer J 3rd. Reconstructed mandibular defects: fibula free flaps and osseointegrated implants. Plast Reconstr Surg. 1997;99:356–65.
16. Rohner D, Bucher P, Kunz C, Hammer B, Schenk RK, Prein J. Treatment of severe atrophy of the maxilla with the prefabricated free vascularized fibula flap. Clin Oral Implants Res. 2002;13:44–52.
17. Bertossi D, Bissolotti G, Corrocher G, Anesi A, Nocini PF. O.301 The use of tapered dental implants in severe jaw atrophies. J Craniomaxillofac Surg. 2008;36(Suppl1):S76. https://doi.org/10.1016/S1010-5182(08)71425-2.
18. Hakim SG, Kimmerle H, Trenkle T, Sieg P, Jacobsen HC. Masticatory rehabilitation following upper and lower jaw reconstruction using vascularised free fibula flap and enossal implants—19 years of experience with a comprehensive concept. Clin Oral Investig. 2015;19:525–34.
19. Chang YM, Chan CP, Shen YF, Wei FC. Soft tissue management using palatal mucosa around endosteal implants in vascularized composite grafts in the mandible. Int J Oral Maxillofac Surg. 1999;28:341–3.
20. Artzi Z, Tai H, Moses O, Kozlovsky A. Mucosal considerations for osseointegrated implants. J Prosthet Dent. 1993;40:427–32.
21. Bedrossian E, Gongloff RK. Considerations in placement of implants through existing split-thickness skin graft vestibuloplasty. A case report. Int J Oral Maxillofac Implants. 1990;5:401–4.
22. Newman MG, Flemmig TE. Periodontal considerations of implants and implant-associated microbiota. J Dent Educ. 1988;52:737–44.
23. Tsai CY, Ueda M, Hata K-I, Horie K, Hibino Y, Sugimura Y, et al. Clinical results of cultured epithelial cell grafting in the oral and maxillofacial region. J Craniomaxillofac Surg. 1997;25:4–8.
24. Hayter JP, Cawood JI. Oral rehabilitation with endosteal implants and free flaps. Int J Oral Maxillofac Surg. 1996;25:3–12.
25. Ten Bruggenkaa CM, K Ler G. Palatal mucosa grafts for dental implant devices. Oral Surg. 1991;72:154–8.
26. Chiapasco M, Biglioli F, Autelitano L, Romeo E, Brusati R. Clinical outcome of dental implants placed in fibula-free flaps used for the reconstruction of maxillomandibular defects following ablation for tumors or osteoradionecrosis. Clin Oral Implants Res. 2006;17:220–8.
27. Kumar VV, Jacob PC, Kekatpure V, Hedne N, Koch FP, Kuriakose MA. The Jugaad technique for jaw reconstruction: denture based inverse planning. J Maxillofac Oral Surg. 2016;15:346–8.
28. Anesi A, Bissolotti G, Toller N, Corrocher G, Chiarini L, Nocini PF. O.322 Ameloblastic flbroma in a 6-year-old child: case report. J Craniomaxillofac Surg. 2008;36(Suppl1):S81. https://doi.org/10.1016/S1010-5182(08)71446-X.
29. Anesi A, Albanese M, Gerosa R, Corrocher G, Gambarini G, Nocini PF. Mandibular ameloblastic fibroma in 6-years-old girl: a case report. Minerva Stomatol. 2008;57(10):549–55. English, Italian.

The manufacturer's authorised representative in the EU is Springer
Nature Customer Service Centre GmbH, Europaplatz 3, 69115 Heidelberg,
Germany. If you have any concerns regarding our products, please
contact ProductSafety@springernature.com

Printed and bound by CPI Group (UK) Ltd, Croydon, CR0 4YY
22/09/2026
02221077-0002